"In *Kigo*, Lorie Dechar gifts us h⟨...⟩ ⟨...⟩nese medicine. Nature and spirit are ravelled through this beautiful work and Lorie is our perceptive guide through the seasons. She unfolds the Chinese characters to pluck wisdom from their embedded symbols, inspiring practitioners to draw on their own inner resources to match the majesty of the points."

—*John Kirkwood, author of* The Way of the Five
Elements *and* The Way of the Five Seasons

"*Kigo* brings to life the wisdom, spirit and poetry embedded in the names of the acupuncture points. This book will be of value for practitioners of Chinese medicine, Qigong and other healing modalities that recognize the movement of Qi through the meridians of the body. Lorelei Chang's original calligraphy adds to the beauty and magic of the text."

—*Robert Peng, author of* The Master Key: Qigong
Secrets for Vitality, Love, and Wisdom

"Lorie Dechar draws on an impressively wide range of Chinese and other sources to bring the 'spirit' of many acupuncture points to life. She also relies on her years of experience as a practitioner to reveal how points can be used to bring about a profound change in a person's spirit."

—*Peter Mole, M.A., Lic.Ac., M.B.AC.C., Dean of College of
Integrated Chinese Medicine, Reading, UK, and co-author
of* Five Element Constitutional Acupuncture

"Both practical and magical, this book is a beautiful addition to the pantheon of commentaries on acupuncture. With gentle poetry and deep experience, Lorie brings alive the healing that happens in each of us whether we are giving or receiving acupuncture. Just open and read any page as a salve for the spirit or pithy instructions that will be just right."

—*Josephine K. Spilka, M.S., L.Ac.*

"Rarely, and only if we are lucky, we find ourselves in the presence of a human being who truly changes our life, and maybe even our perception of life. That happened in 2010 when I found myself, accidentally, in a three-day workshop with Lorie Dechar. This book is the culmination of years of inspirational work, setting out new possibilities, so enjoy every word, as her heart just might be speaking directly to yours..."

—*Jen Wade, Joint Principal, The Acupuncture Academy*

KIGO

Exploring the Spiritual Essence of Acupuncture Points Through the Changing Seasons

LORIE EVE DECHAR

ILLUSTRATIONS BY LORIE EVE DECHAR

CALLIGRAPHY BY LORELEI CHANG

FOREWORD BY RANDINE LEWIS

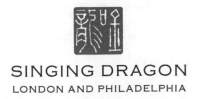

SINGING DRAGON

LONDON AND PHILADELPHIA

First published in Great Britain in 2021 by Singing Dragon,
an imprint of Jessica Kingsley Publishers
An Hachette Company

1

Copyright © Lorie Eve Dechar 2021
Illustrations copyright © Lorie Eve Dechar 2021
Calligraphy copyright © Lorelei Chang 2021
Foreword copyright © Randine Lewis 2021

Cover artwork: Lorie Eve Dechar

Epigraph from *The Narrow Road to the Deep North, and Other Travel Sketches*
by Matsuo Basho, translated by Nobuyuki Yuasa. Copyright © Nobuyuki
Yausa, 1966. Reproduced by kind permission of Penguin Random House.

A CIP catalogue record for this title is available from the
British Library and the Library of Congress

ISBN 978 1 78775 256 6
eISBN 978 1 78775 257 3

Printed and bound by CPI Group (UK) Ltd, Croydon, CR0 4YY

Jessica Kingsley Publishers' policy is to use papers that are natural,
renewable and recyclable products and made from wood grown in
sustainable forests. The logging and manufacturing processes are expected
to conform to the environmental regulations of the country of origin.

Jessica Kingsley Publishers
73 Collier Street
London N1 9BE, UK

www.singingdragon.com

What is important is to keep our mind high in the world of true understanding, and returning to the world of our daily experience to seek therein the truth of beauty. No matter what we may be doing at a given moment, we must not forget that it has a bearing upon our everlasting self which is poetry.

MATSUO BASHO

Contents

Foreword

The things I value most in life I came across serendipitously. Chinese medicine was one of these. Meeting Lorie Dechar was another.

After studying Western medicine, I fell in love with the poetic philosophy of the *Tao*. While I couldn't wrap my mind around it, Chinese medicine had a profound effect on something deep inside that conventional medicine couldn't touch. Its healing power deeply changed me and the trajectory my life was to take. I opened a clinic, wrote a book, began speaking and offering healing retreats. I was on fire watching others heal through the power of this amazing medicine while burning myself out trying to help them. Overdosing on my frantic *yang* pursuits, it seemed I was the one needing help.

A few weeks later, I found myself lying on a carpeted floor at Esalen Institute, covered by cushions, pillows and a desperately needed heaviness provided by our retreat facilitator. It felt as though this part of me that needed to prove itself through overworking needed to die or it would take me over like a cancer. An ancient burial ritual was enacted, calling on the power of the Taoist Queen Mother of the West, who presided over my "death," as the deep, dark heaviness of Earth absorbed my overdoing. This was my introduction to Lorie Dechar, a true master of the soft power of *yin*, so often neglected in our medicine, using the stuff of life to transform pain and trauma into healing. She was orchestrating real live alchemy on the spot, and I honestly felt reborn.

I had recently come across Lorie's *Five Spirits*,[1] whose words reached deep into my soul with the same ancient and profound wisdom that brought me into acupuncture in the first place. I had to find this powerhouse. And, coincidentally, she happened to be hosting a retreat during the exact time I could go. Her presence changed my relationship with the medicine, and many years later, I daresay she's gotten even stronger.

Mastery can come in many ways. While our left brains are impressed by acupuncture's ability to quantify specifically defined healing goals and repeat them, its true heart resides in its artistry. Here, the artist, empty even of intention, unleashes a mysterious unseen power, and healing happens. Few are those like Lorie Dechar who can spontaneously harness this therapeutic power.

Throughout this book, masterfully woven words wrap you up in the poetry of the Orient's original healing magic. Like my ancient burial ritual, each conveys a story that rings true to the timeless store of wisdom we all carry within.

As I read *Kigo: Exploring the Spiritual Essence of Acupuncture Points Through the Changing Seasons*, I linger in the felt experience of each point until I absorb it, or it absorbs me. I'm not sure which. I am transported to the sacred mountains of the East. And as always happens when Lorie transmits this healing power, I am changed by her words. A gateway opens up in a landscape where my soul feels at home, and I'm left with a fresh remembrance of a secret knowing I've always had but couldn't quite access. I am renewed. May these words open up the same portal in you as you begin to remember the true healing power of this ancient wisdom, and let it ignite the master within.

RANDINE LEWIS, Ph.D., L.Ac., FABORM
Author of *The Infertility Cure* and *The Way of the Fertile Soul*

Acknowledgments

There is no doubt in my mind that it has "taken a village" to bring this book from its first blink of inspiration into actual, manifest form. Five years ago, while running along a dirt road on a wild, rainy November afternoon, I was head-struck by a falling bit of starlight! Out of the blue, I made the connection between a "kigo"—the special season word that potentizes the Japanese haiku—and the spark of spirit hidden in the acupuncture point. After my run, I sat down on a chair by the window in my office, looked out at the rushing gray clouds and falling leaves, and wrote the first point poem. The star spark took root and since then this book has had a determined life of its own!

Many hands have helped with the word weaving. Threads extend through my local support network, my friends, as well as the natural environment of Blue Hill, Maine. They extend globally to my community of students, colleagues and patients who engage in the work of Alchemical Healing. There are far too many of you to name here but you know who you are, and I love and appreciate you with all my Heart.

There are, however, a few people who have directly contributed to the production of this book whom I want to especially acknowledge. First, Claire Wilson, my London editor at Singing Dragon, who spotted the electronic proposal I submitted through the web portal, saw its potential and valiantly pitched the project to the acquisitions committee at Jessica Kingsley Publishers. Thanks to Maddy

Budd, editorial assistant extraordinaire and my reliable personal advisor throughout the process, as well as to production editor Victoria Peters, copyeditor Bonnie Craig, proofreader Katherine Laidler, and typesetter Rosamund Bird, who brought their dedication to quality to the final polishing of the manuscript. It has been a delight and an honor to work with this dedicated team of women.

Next, I thank my New York copy editor, Charlotte Kelly, who did a masterful job of editing the draft manuscript and preparing it for submission. Charlotte, I could not have done it without you! Only someone who has combed through hundreds of pages of text containing English, *pinyin*, Chinese medical terminology, a multitude of Chinese characters and dozens of footnotes can have any idea of the effort it takes to edit this kind of manuscript. I am blown away by the care, patience, persistence and precision—and I would add good humor—Charlotte brought to the project.

Next, a bow of gratitude to two acupuncturist sinologists and researchers who especially inspired me in the writing of this book: Debra Kaatz, whose book *Characters of Wisdom: Taoist Tales of the Acupuncture Points* is a treasure trove of poetic scholarship, and Dominique Hertzer, whose translation of the *Xiuzhen Tu* (The Chart of the Cultivation of Ultimate Reality) and lecture at the Second Annual TCM Kongress in Denmark in September 2009 encouraged me to look further into the mythology of the Taoist spirit animals.

I also want to acknowledge spirit dancer, healer and artist, Lorelei Chang, who graces these pages with the flowing brush strokes of her calligraphy.

I place flowers at the feet of the many mountain poets, radical wanderers and landscape painters whose footsteps I follow.

Last, first and everywhere in between, I thank Benjamin

Fox, my alchemical partner, teacher, star sibling, husband and friend, who has put up with, cajoled, critiqued, complimented and inspired my creativity and, most of all, somehow continued to love me through it all.

Author's Note

Over the centuries, innumerable attempts have been made to standardize the translation and spelling of Chinese terms presented in Western texts. However, there is still no universally accepted way of handling this task. In coming to my own decisions, I have based my choices on four variables: clarity, scholarship, familiarity and respect.

Romanization

The modern, more familiar *pinyin* form of Romanization will be used throughout the book.

Capitalization

I have chosen to follow the lead of my first teacher, Professor J. R. Worsley, and capitalize the names of the elements, seasons and points, as well as the names of the organs or officials presiding over the meridians, to emphasize that we are using these words in a special way that is different from ordinary English and Western medical usage.

Italicization

Chinese terms are italicized and lower case. With compound terms (where two or more characters, known as radicals, come together to form a single word), I leave spaces between the two or more italicized Chinese words—i.e. Lung 1 - Middle Palace - *Zhong Fu*—so that it is easier to grasp the relationship to the two or more radicals that compose the character.

Chinese words that are commonly used in English, such as *qi, yin* and *yang,* are italicized the first time and non-italicized moving forward, as are certain foreign words that are central to the text, such as kigo and haiku.

Characters

I include the graphics of the Chinese character names for each point. I have learned a great deal from spending time studying and tracing the lines of these ancient characters. Each one contains an element of wisdom that cannot be totally grasped through the intellect alone. I encourage readers to take time to meditate on the characters themselves as another way to glean the spiritual essence of the points presented in these pages.

Introduction

Kigo: Season Word

Kigo means "season word" in Japanese. A kigo is a word or phrase traditionally associated with a particular time of year. Like a single perfect brush stroke in a Japanese landscape painting, a kigo gives us a glimpse of the ephemeral spirit that imbues each moment of the turning year. Last cricket song, sickle moon, light snow on crimson maple leaves, cherry blossoms, fireflies, paper lanterns rustling in the wind—the host of associations, feelings and memories that these words evoke in us allow for the potency and economy of expression that are the hallmark of the most famous form of Japanese poetry, the three-line *haiku*. In her essay *Kigo and Form*, poet Kiyoko Tokutomi describes kigo as the "window of the haiku."[2] It is the word that takes us beyond the black-and-white letters of the text into the sensuous living world of the poem.

Although the idea of kigo is in some ways uniquely Japanese, there is a universal resonance to these kinds of words. For all humans, the turning of the seasons has a profound effect on health, emotions and states of mind, as well as the divinities we celebrate and the ways we relate to ourselves and to the world around us. Kigo words sing to us because of the intrinsic connection between language, the atmospheres and rhythms of the natural world and our own bodies and souls. The words we use create the world we experience; the world we experience profoundly affects the choices we make, the possibilities we envision and the way we live our lives.

Through the deft weaving of kigo words, the great Japanese haiku poets astonish us into remembering *mono no aware*— the "Ah!-ness of things." In the following pages, I call on the power of the kigo to remind us of the "Ah!-ness" of the healing encounter and to re-enliven our spiritual connection to the acupuncture points, the *zhang fu* organs and the meridians of traditional Chinese medicine. Most point directories focus on the points' anatomical locations, their functions and the physical symptoms they can be used to treat. But our interest is elsewhere. Here, we look to discover how inserting a needle at the right moment into the right point can open a window to a person's soul, taking us beyond the surface of the session deep into a person's inner world, the way a well-chosen kigo opens us to the heart and soul of the haiku.

At the center of every point is *wu* 無 emptiness into which *shen* 神 spirit can be called. In order to enter this space of infinite possibility, this space of *wu* emptiness, we must first let go of our comfortable attitude of "already knowing" the limits of what an acupuncture point can do. When we bring an awakened awareness, devotion and not knowing to our encounter with the point—whether through a needle, a moxa cone, a touch, a flower essence, an essential oil or an image— our presence becomes an incantation. Through this special kind of receptivity, sight and awareness, we transform the point from a number on a line or a sensitized spot on the skin to a mystery—a doorway into a process of psycho-spiritual transformation.

A Brief Introduction to the Five Elements

This book is divided into five parts. Each part is related to one of the five seasons that are recognized in Five Element Acupuncture: Winter, Spring, Summer, Late Summer and Autumn. In Five Element Acupuncture, each of these seasons is associated with a specific Element, vegetative cycle, color, sound, emotion, spirit and set of acupuncture meridians and points. Each season is also related to transits of life, to our experience of being human and to kigo—words, images and atmospheres that gather up the essence of the spiritual dimension of that particular time of year.

For the ancient Taoist physicians and sages who developed many of the most important theories and practices of traditional Chinese medicine, nature is not only the physical matrix of our being but the doorway through which the mystery of *Tao* 道 the Divine path or Way of the Cosmos manifests as a reality in our lives. Spirit is not "far away in Heaven" but here, now and visible in the world around us. It is only through devoted attention to the natural world, through a direct encounter with the wisdom of nature, that we can come anywhere close to knowing the unknowable Tao and grasping the essence of an embodied spiritual experience of life.

In the Taoist theory of *wu xing* 五行, the Five Elements reflect the ancient understanding that Tao is related to the macrocosm of nature and to the microcosm of an individual human being. *Wu xing* describes the cycle of transformation inherent to all carbon-based life. I have looked long and hard over three decades of practice and have yet to discover a process or system that does not in some way follow this pattern of gestation, growth, blossoming, fruition and decline (and round again). In every organic process, in every being with a soul, the round of the seasons and the cyclic intermingling of the basic Elements—Water, Wood, Fire, Earth and Metal— metaphorically and practically describe the processes of change in life on our planet.

The Five Element Wheel is a mandala, an expression of unity in diversity, a geometric pattern that gives us a glimpse of the Divine order of the universe. It is a symbol of the self, the wholeness of an individual personality, the authentic impulse to become "me" that is at the core of every human life. Our lives are an expression of this cosmic wheel as we move from the initiating impulse of Wood, through the maturation of Fire, the ripening of Earth, the letting go of Metal and the deep rest and regeneration of Water. Again and again, the Wheel turns and we turn with it.

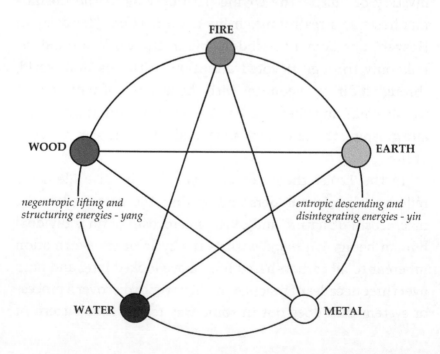

WU XING: FIVE ELEMENT WHEEL

The Points

With the proper attitude and vision, the acupuncture points become doorways that allow us to access the potent energies of the seasons and elements at pivotal moments in a person's life. The points have the capacity to bring us closer to our own wholeness, to invite spirit and soul back into relationship with the body. They are catalysts to alchemical processes that initiate change, enhance vision, support intention, help us to bear chaos and uncertainty and, ultimately, to manifest our Tao.

In order to bring this kind of potency to the points, we need to care deeply about them, to take time to know them and be friends with them. We need to reflect on their meaning, listen for their hidden poetry, understand their individual medicine and touch them with reverence. It is my experience and my firm belief that only through our ongoing "befriending" of them will the points reveal their full spiritual potency.

This book is not meant to be a how-to manual but something more like a letter of introduction to some of my most beloved friends, a series of meditations on time and place and the mysterious healing of the soul. In these pages, I share experiences with points that have spoken to me, ones that I have come to know intimately over many years of practice. Each point offering begins with the meridian point number, name in English and *pinyin* (the most widely accepted form of Romanized Chinese), followed by the traditional Chinese character. Next, I offer a haiku, a poem I have written to honor the gifts I have received from the point, as well as the *kairos*, the particular time of the season or uniquely decisive moment, that I feel captures the point's essence.

In the commentaries, I discuss my sense of the points' nature and spirit and some of the methods I have found most useful in waking up their spiritual potency, including specific essential oils, flower essences and needle and moxibustion techniques. In some cases, I include brief descriptions of remarkable clinical moments when the point activated a shift, a transformational experience of "Ah!-ness" in the treatment room.

Beyond the joy of sharing my clinical experiences from over 30 years of practice and my gratitude and love for the mystery and beauty of this medicine, my hope is that this book will inspire you to re-envision and deepen your relationship to the points. I encourage you to spend time with the points, tools and meditations, but please do not limit yourself to the points explored here! Every point on the body has its own magic and mystery. The ultimate goal of this book is to support you in creating your own spirit point palette and activating the deeper spiritual resonance of any point you choose to use in your own practice.

Hundreds of thousands of acupuncturists, whether practicing today or centuries before, have cured countless physical, emotional and spiritual problems without even knowing the specific names of the points they may be using. By needling certain points in combination with others, recommending various herbal tonics and maintaining a clarity of intention, commitment and a simple depth of care, much healing can be achieved. What I am proposing is that the kind of conscious, intentional work with the spirit of the points that I describe here can be effectively and powerfully interwoven with other forms of acupuncture. This results in a kind of psychological or soul-level healing that is completely compatible with the ancient traditions of Chinese medicine. It's also particularly valuable to Westerners, who are often stuck in chronic states of abstract psychic distress, alienated from the rhythm, beauty and poetry of the natural world and from their own authentic being.

Although the points reside at specific locations and are embedded in the fibers of our skin, they have the capacity to affect infinite and transcendent aspects of our being. Even without needles, we can use words, touch, oils and flower essences to open others and ourselves to these transcendent realms. We can use these tools in our everyday life as well as in the treatment room to heal ourselves, each other and the soul of our world.

A Note on Placebo

While the names, locations and indications for the points have been discussed in Chinese medical texts for over 2000 years, it has not yet been proven to the satisfaction of rational Western science and medicine that the points actually exist as a physiological reality. Despite decades of studies, no one has yet been able to prove without a doubt that stimulating these points with needles, moxa or pressure has any predictable, reliable effect on specific symptoms. For those looking to place acupuncture firmly in the fold of modern scientific medicine, these doubts pose a significant problem.

However, for those more interested in discovering what traditional Chinese healers were actually up to in their explorations, modern double-blind studies and statistical assessments are of less concern. For acupuncturists and other practitioners who wish to plumb the depths of this tradition in order to discover a new, more generous and expansive way of approaching healing, it is more important to try to understand the medicine from within its own language, logic and imagery. For those of us who have even once seen color, light and presence return to a patient's eyes when the needle touches the spirit at the center of the point, the search for a new consciousness that can contain and give language to this level of experience becomes the primary concern.

But there is one rich area of recent Western medical investigation that is quite relevant to our conversation: the growing field of placebo studies. Here the lines that Western science has so carefully drawn between the mind and the body, between thought, belief and physical function, are beginning to blur. As we delve deeper into the mystery of the placebo effect, the worldviews of Western allopathic and traditional Chinese medicine are finding common ground. Using randomized trial studies and real-time brain magnetic resonance imaging, researchers at Harvard Medical School, the National Institutes of Health and elsewhere are discovering that the words we use, the attitudes we bring and even the thoughts we think during an encounter with a patient have a definite and profound impact on physiology and the outcome of treatment.

Placebo is defined in the West as an inactive medicine or substance administered by a doctor. Typically for a Western physician, this could be a deactivated sugar pill or aspirin, but it could also include a word of encouragement, a positive affirmation, the well-timed return of a phone call or a potent image. The word *placebo* comes from the Latin, *I shall please*, and points to the Western medical idea that a substance is being administered to please a patient without any real belief in its efficacy. Until recently in Western medicine, placebo had a negative connotation and was considered a way to soothe, placate or even trick a patient into paying for something that the doctor believes has no value. Because of this, the placebo effect—the capacity of "medically inactive" words or substances to support recovery and healing—

has been regarded with extreme distrust, and efforts have been taken to eliminate it as a possible influence in the clinical encounter.

However, when we turn to the Chinese character for the word placebo, we discover a different underlying attitude. The Chinese word *an wei ji* 安慰剂 is made up of three separate radicals. *An* 安 is a picture of a woman relaxing comfortably under the roof of a house. Used alone, the word means to calm or set one's mind at ease. *Wei* 慰 is a picture that indicates a soothing cloth over the radical for Heart. It means to calm, console, comfort and express sympathy. *Ji* 剂 is the radical for neatly and evenly prepared, next to a picture of a knife. This word indicates a portion or dose of medicine.

In considering the Chinese character, we recognize the understanding that placebos have the capacity to console and comfort, to smooth the upsets of the Heart and to function as powerful medicine. The character does not include the West's negative connotation of deception and unwarranted personal gain. From the Chinese perspective, the comforting and consoling aspect of the practitioner–patient relationship is neither extraneous nor questionable. Because the mental, emotional and physical aspects of illness are not held as separate, healing initiated through the practitioner–patient relationship is considered a critical part of the process—at times an even more important factor than the chemistry of the drugs, the placement of the needle or even the exact nature of the therapy.

When we turn to the Chinese character for medicine *yao* 药, we discover a picture of 纟 silk threads and 勺 the spoon used by the physician to administer the dose to the patient. Silk threads in a Chinese character imply the idea of connection, weaving and binding. So the meaning implicit in the character for medicine includes the idea of a binding together, an engaged connection between physician and patient. And when we consider the spoon, we must also consider the hand that holds it. The power is not just in the medicine, the needle, the oil or the flower essence but also in the hand, Heart and vision of the practitioner who chooses and offers it.

Modern Western science is proving what Chinese doctors and other traditional healers have understood through empirical observation for thousands of years.

- There is a connection between doctor and patient— silk threads that bind them together in the healing process. The efficacy of treatment is impacted by their relationship.

- The rituals or formal acts embedded in the clinical encounter, the authority of the practitioner and context of the therapy matter. Positive beliefs about future outcomes may trigger those outcomes.

- How big the practitioner draws the circle defines the territory the patient will explore.

Healing does not always involve a chemical or biological intervention. It can sometimes arise from a shift in attitude or belief and accompanying changes in the patient's neurochemistry and physiology as well as in their soul. In Western scientific terms, it may result from the spontaneous activation of key neural pathways in the brain resulting in dopamine and endogenous opiate release. And in the words of 2000-year-old Chinese medical text the *Neijing Suwen*, healing can be the result of "transmitting the Essence and invoking the gods,"[3] whether with a needle, a moxa cone, a visionary encounter or a word.

It is not in any way my intention to suggest that the points work only through the effect of placebo. Touching, breathing and living with these points with patients over decades, I have absolutely no doubt that correct stimulation of the points induces real physiological changes on endocrinal, muscular and neurological levels along with profound shifts on the level of the emotions and psyche. What I am suggesting is that traditional Chinese doctors first understood that how we speak to our patients, the connections we make, the images we call on and the subtle energies we touch have a huge impact on the outcome of treatment.

The Subtle Body

Between another and myself, there is an unknown universe. The acupuncture point can be a doorway to this domain. As we insert the needle into *wu*—the whirling emptiness at the center of the vortex of the point—a field of possibility constellates as Earth and Heaven join together in my body. Like lotus blossoms opening their petals on an infinite sea, the points beckon to us to rediscover the ephemeral spirit hidden at the heart of the material world. They invite us back to ourselves and to an enlivened encounter with another. Most of all, they call us forward toward healing that includes the beauty, creativity, uncertainty, courage and passion that are the hallmarks of a truly healthy human life.

The Seasons

Water: Winter Season

"Water brings us closest to Tao." Over 2000 years ago, the philosopher-poet Lao Tzu wrote these words as he contemplated the movement of life in the world around him. "Water," he said, "knows how to benefit all things without striving with them."[1] It goes without resistance to the low, dark and hidden places feared by others. Continuing Lao Tzu's meditation on the Water Element, we experience Water's seamless shape-shifting as it transforms from solid to liquid to gas, from rock-hard structure to impalpable vapor, from placid surface to chaotic vortices, from passive receptivity to activating power, from oceanic depths to the heights of sunlit geysers. We see that Water embodies the *yin/yang* paradox of *qi*—the life force itself—as it maintains its intrinsic identity through its infinite varieties of expression. Moving in accord with its own nature yet changing endlessly in response to the conditions it encounters, the Water Element embodies the mystery of Tao, the Divine wisdom of the cosmos. The Water Element lives in us not only in the pulsating fluids of our spinal column and brain, our bone marrow, sexual fluids, hormones, lymph and blood but also in our souls.

The Chinese character for the Water Element is *shui* 水. It represents a picture of meandering currents. The flowing nature of the Element is graphically expressed in the character.

In traditional Chinese medicine, the Water Element is related to the season of Winter. It represents the time of year when the force of life and the energy to sustain it must be carefully stored and treasured. In winter, the fallen seeds and decomposed micronutrients of the Metal season are buried beneath the snow. In the womb of the soil, life waits in a state of nearly inert stillness, gestating and gathering strength as it prepares for re-emergence.

On the Five Element Wheel, we find Water opposite Metal at the bottom of the cycle. This affirms our understanding of Water's tendency to flow down toward the yin, dark, cool and receptive. But unlike Metal, which we find on the entropic right, yin, downward-directed side of the Wheel, Water sits at the bottom of the negentropic left side of the Wheel. Here, at the lowest point of the growth cycle, life is infused with the yang, upsurging energies of spirit and renewal that rise from the depths of the underworld. At the heart of darkness, after the life force has descended to the roots and bulbs of plants, to the underground springs, the bear caves and bones, there is a quickening, a turning. In mid-winter, as snow falls, ice cracks and the temperatures plummet, the morning light grows brighter, the days grow longer and deep within the Wood, the sap begins to rise.

With Water, we come to understand that the elements and the seasons are not static things. Rather they are symbolic expressions of change and movement through time. Winter begins when the yin has gathered to its fullest extent, in an atmosphere tinged with the minor-key longing and grief of Metal. But by the time we reach Water season's close, the yang qi is on the rise and the world begins to vibrate with the brightening chords of Wood's brash and hopeful exuberance.

And in between the symphony of winter plays on in the swirling snow clouds, the whining winds and the pale notes of sparrows pecking dry cones beneath the cedar trees.

Kigo words evoke the mysterious duality of Water, its depth, stillness, harshness and perseverance and also its potency, spontaneity and surprising vitality. Frost flowers on fallen birch leaves, diamond-bright stars in a black night, cold hands warmed by a meager fire, a red-tailed hawk flying hungry above a snow-covered field, ice on the bay and early darkness. Water calls us to accept the reality of danger, the difficulty of survival as well as nature's necessary culling of the weak. Yet it also offers us the possibility of restoration and depth and the gifts of courage, resilience and wisdom.

Vegetative Expression

During the cold of the Winter season, the qi and sap descend to the roots of plants where life forces are gathered, stored, protected and infused with new vitality. The seed is the vegetative archetype of storage and preserving, which are primary functions of this Element. Now the hard seeds rest, unmoving, in the darkness. But this time of yin hibernation and gestation is ultimately a regeneration of the life force that opens the way for the vigorous upward surging of early Spring.

Deep in winter, the sap stirs in the unseen roots of the trees. At the heart of the seed, desire stirs. And as the Wheel turns from Water to Wood, the moment comes when the seed splits, the egg cracks, the water breaks and birth becomes imperative. Then, the stored qi is liberated to fuel new growth as the "I Am" of Water turns to the "I Become" of Wood.

Color/Sound/Odor/Emotion

The Color of Water is Blue/Black

In the *Neijing Suwen*, we read, "Blue/black is the color of the North, it pervades the kidneys and opens the two lower orifices and retains the essential substances within the kidneys."[2] To diagnose the health of the Water Element, look at the sides of the eyes, temples and laugh lines around the mouth for a range from pale summer sky to blue-black ocean depths. The *Neijing Suwen* tells us, "When they are black like coal they are without life... When they are black like the wings of a crow they are full of life."[3] Study blue and black in nature. Study them in both balance and imbalance and notice how your Heart responds. Bring this feeling with you into the treatment room.

The Sound is Groan

Listen for a voice that seeks the lowest places, that tends downward toward rest and even hiddenness, especially at the end of sentences, or a groan that sounds gravelly, like water running across pebbles in a shallow stream.

The Odor is Putrid

Smell for something a bit sharp and salty, like the beach at low tide or New York City subway steps early on Sunday morning.

The Emotion is Fear

This can manifest as frozen paralysis and contraction but also hyper-reactive fight or flight. However, fear transforms into courage, so Water may also be the bravest of the elements.

The Officials

Water is related to the organs of the Kidneys and Bladder. It has to do with the health and vitality of the urogenital system. The Water Element regulates the filtration, distillation and excretion of fluids, the waxing and waning of our sexuality and our capacity to store and wisely mobilize our *jing* 精, our ancestral inherited life essences. Water is a paradox. It supports us not only in our yin need for deeply restorative silence and rest but also, through the adrenal glands that cap the Kidneys, in our yang need to activate our most high-grade fight-or-flight survival drives in the face of threat or danger. To further amplify our understanding of Water's paradoxical twoness of nature, we look to the anatomy of the Kidneys and see that it is the only *zhang fu* organ that is a twin. Two completely separate, independently functioning partners— one right and one left, one yang and one yin—mirror each other at the base of the spine, the firing point of the tailbone, the root of the nervous system, on either side of Governing Vessel 4 - The Gate of Life - *Ming Men*.

The Bladder Official holds the office of Controller of Water Storage. This official is in charge not only of maintaining adequate reserves of fluids and energy but also of maintaining the purity and quality of these reserves and discharging the waste products that result from the filtering role of the Kidney Official. The fact that the Bladder meridian is the longest meridian in the entire body reminds us of the scope of the Bladder's crucial role. Without its capacity for storing and providing fluids for the whole body, no other physical or psychological functions could occur. Through fostering the fluidity and vitality of our bodies, minds and spirits, the Bladder Official "makes the movement and growth of all the other officials possible, and by the presence of the reserves which it controls this official guarantees them security and their future."[4]

The Chinese word for Bladder is *pang guang* 膀 胱, which literally translates as "wing of light." The character contains within it the radicals *rou* 肉 flesh and *guang* 光 light. This character reminds us of Water's role of bringing light and spirit down into matter. The Bladder's appropriate preservation and control of the essences illuminates our being with wisdom and allows us to make good use of the resources we are born with in addition to those that come to us throughout the course of our lives.

The Kidney Official holds the office of Controller of the Waterways and is responsible for the filtration of toxins and impurities and the dispersal of Water to every part of the organism. It controls the separation of Water and qi and moves fluids through the whole body. Also known as the creator of bone and marrow, it is particularly associated with the lumbar spine and brain. It opens the ears and has a significant effect on the reproductive and sexual organs. In some texts, the left *shao yang* aspect where yang rises from yin is named "Kidney" but the right *shao yin* aspect where yin descends from yang relates to the Water's capacity to manifest Tao and is called *ming men* 命 门 door of destiny.

We see that this official has more hidden and less physical responsibilities. Beyond its functions of Water filtration, dispersal and storage, it is responsible for the storage of *jing*—the fluid seed of life and genetic memory passed from one generation to the next. Through the storage, protection and appropriate dispersal of *jing*, the Kidney Official guards our life force and is a determining factor in our ability to live in accordance with our authentic Tao or destiny.

Zhi: The Spirit of Water

The spirit of the Water Element is the *zhi* 志 translated as "will" or "ambition." The *Neijing Suwen* tells us that Water "is of the north and the creatures of the north are scaled... fish, reptiles, snakes."[5] The Chinese character *bei* 北 north is a picture of two people standing back to back. It reminds us that Water is related to our spine, to our back, to the unseen, primal, instinctual, non-verbal aspects of our nervous system. The Bladder meridian, which follows the course of the lumbar and thoracic vertebrae, connects us neurologically to our earliest vertebrate ancestors, the water-born reptiles who made the first journey from sea to land many millions of years ago. This connection to the back, the spine and the primal nervous system offers a clue to the nature of Water's spirit and points to the link between the *zhi*, the spirit of the Water Element, and the deeply embedded ancient knowing of our primal "reptilian brain."[6]

The *zhi* is the guardian of the *jing* or inherited essences that fuel our instincts as well as our capacity to accumulate wisdom over time. It is like the pilot light, the spark that ignites our will to become and to manifest our authentic nature. The *zhi* is related to the First Chakra and the collective unconscious. It regulates our sexuality, our survival drives, our long-term ancestral memories and our inherited wisdom. It is responsible for the balancing of fear and courage, fight, freeze and flight.

Ultimately, it is through working internally with the potent, high-grade energies of the *zhi* that we gain wisdom and an embodied connection to the Divine. In the sacred mountain that is the symbol of the self, the *zhi* is the lower spirit that resides at the very bottom of the underground labyrinths and passageways. At the core of being, in the depths of the pelvis of our bodies and our planet, we find the natural home of the *zhi* spirit. Here, the downward trajectory of Water reverses to become a phosphorescent upsurge, the bubbling sulfur spring of the underworld. Dreaming becomes desire, the seed case cracks, the sprout emerges and we are catapulted back from darkness into life.

Water's spirit question: Is my personal will in integrity with my time, my age, my Tao?

Spirit Animal: The Two-Headed Deer

The spirit of the Kidneys looks like a Two-Headed Deer. Its name is Mystic Darkness and its color is *xuan* 玄 black, so dark as to be nearly invisible. Although it cannot be seen with the ordinary eyes, Mystic Darkness can be seen with the eyes of the Heart, in the white mist of early morning or the gray clouds of twilight, when the vulnerable and easily frightened creature feels safe enough to emerge from hiding.

Along with its spirit name, the Two-Headed Deer has a given name: To Nourish the Infant. This second name refers to the Kidney's association with sexuality and the activation of sexual fluids in service of the creation of new life. But it also refers to the function of the *zhi* in the appropriate regulation of the use of *jing*, not only in the passage of essences from one generation to the next through physical birth but also in the initiation, gestation and cultivation of the life of the spiritual embryo hidden in the *dan tian* 丹田 cinnabar field— the alchemical vessel of our bodies. This second function of the Two-Headed Deer is what allows it to become the nourishing spirit of destiny.

The Two-Headed Deer is a creature of opposites. It is yin and yang. It sees both dark and light, and its two heads look in opposite directions. One head looks to the past of our ancestors and the karmic influences that inform our current situation. The other looks to the future of our children and the nature of the legacy we will leave behind according to how we bring our will to bear on our life force. Holding the key to both memory and will, the Two-Headed Deer is where past and future meet. The Two-Headed Deer understands that the future is influenced by the past and yet, moment to moment, it is my immediate response to the situations I face that determine whether I am in alignment with my own Tao.

The Two-Headed Deer's favorite food is *ling zhi* 靈 芝 reishi mushroom. This mushroom grows in dark, hidden places in the forest. Its discovery requires patience, keen senses and carefully preserved ancestral memories of its growth habits and whereabouts. It has a potent tonifying effect on the physical organ of the Kidneys. Beyond that, we know that *ling zhi* refers to a special aspect of spirit, something that is fairy-like, soulful, mysterious, tricky and difficult to perceive. The character on the left, *ling* 靈, is a picture of two dancing sorceresses calling the raindrops of the Divine light down from Heaven. The radical on the right, *zi* 芝, combines the part radical *cao* 艹 plant with *zhi* 之, the phonetic that means "of" or "belongs to." So we see that hidden away in the character for *ling zhi*—the herb of the soul—is the clue to Water's medicine: the capacity to call down Heavenly spirit into our embodied life on Earth.

The Two-Headed Deer is the protector of the northern direction. We call on the Two-Headed Deer to support us when we approach the darkness of winter, to accompany us as we travel through the unknown or when we are threatened or paralyzed by fear. The Two-Headed Deer stands at our back and keeps watch over things that are hidden, things we cannot see. She is the protector of the spine and Kidneys and gives us the courage to step into the darkness or to simply rest and wait patiently through the night until the morning light returns.

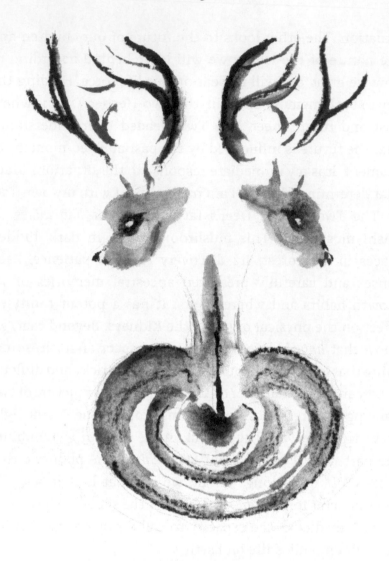

THE TWO-HEADED DEER

Archetype: The Dark Goddess

The Dark Goddess, the Goddess of Life, Death and Rebirth, is the primary archetype of the Water Element. In Taoist mythology, the Dark Goddess is *Xi Wang Mu* 西王 母 the Western Queen Mother. *Xi Wang Mu* resides in the land of the setting sun where she maintains her sovereignty over the darkness of the night. She is sometimes said to live in a cave in the bowels of the Earth below the mythical Kunlun Mountain where she presides over the Yellow Springs— the geysers of the waters of life and death that gush up from the underworld. It is said that "without a whirlwind carriage on feathered wheels, no one can ever reach here."[7] At other times, she is said to dwell in the Garden of the Peach Tree of Immortality located on Pestle Mountain in the Tortoise Mountain Range. Her palace lies in the splendid parks of Kunlun and is described as "twelve storied jade buildings and towers of jasper essence...halls of radiant lucid jade, mysterious terraces, and purple kingfisher cinnabar chambers."[8]

In the second century BC, the poet Ssu-ma Hsiang-ju described *Xi Wang Mu* as a formidable guardian at the gate and also a generous hostess, the donor but also the secret keeper of the elixir of immortality.[9] In this way, she sometimes embodies the qualities of the beneficent Mother who cultivates and preserves life, but at other times she is described as a fearsome hybrid Tiger Woman whose sharp, devouring teeth and dangerous fiery eyes can kill in an instant. Emerging from the depths of Taoist mythology, this goddess represents the essential cosmic principle of yin as the foundation of life, of all that is yielding, fecund and gestating, but also the foundation of death, of all that is annihilating, dissolving and disintegrating. Together with her consort Lord King of the East, master of the yang and the rising sun, the Queen Mother commands the constellations, maintains the continuity of cosmic cycles and is the linking factor between the timelessness of Heaven and the time-bound world of Earth. These two represent the Divine cosmic opposites—yin and yang, Water and Fire—none other than the Tao itself as it moves from non-being into being.

But like all archetypal symbols and myths, there is another even greater mystery embedded in the story of *Xi Wang Mu*. An important clue to her true Divine nature is indicated by her direction. While Water's direction is north, the Queen is found in the west, in the realm of the setting sun, the realm of the Metal Element and of death. In fact, she has been called the Tortoise Mother and the Greatly Wondrous Mother of Metal of Tortoise Mountain.[10]

The Taoist Queen Mother of the West is related to underworld goddesses from various cultures, including the Sumerian Ereshkigal, Anatolian Cybele and the Hawaiian Volcano Goddess Pele. In all her various disguises— grandmother, crone, hag, Baba Yaga, dragon and wise woman—she holds the key to the ultimate unknowns of death and rebirth. We meet the Dark Goddess in the depths of the underworld where compression is so great that the opposites reverse and yang heat and Fire rise from the yin below: blue flames, yellow springs, flaming rivers of molten lava, the cataclysmic push of uterine contractions when the birthing time arrives, sexual desire, the propelling impulse of ambition and the fierce claims of our security drives. Her presence is felt in yang emerging from yin and the irrepressible irruptive potency of life's renewal.

Alchemy: Transforming Will into Wisdom

Crucial to a healthy relationship to Water is the alignment of our individual personal will, our drives, desires and ambitions, with the greater will of Tao. Water asks us to listen deeply to the needs of our being. Yet it also demands that we take heed of our larger destiny as it is revealed through the conditions, people and events we encounter. Rather than wasting precious life essences fighting against the way things are, Water invites us to accept the ever-changing forms of life, to go with the flow and to trust that with every descent, there will be a rising; with every death, there will be a resurrection. At this time of year, it is good to go down and in, to eat warm roots and bone broths, to restore ourselves through sleep and meditation as we wait for the quickening, the first stirrings of the possibilities that gestate in the darkness.

Water Spirit Points

Bladder 1 - Eyes Bright - *Jing Ming*

睛明

Late winter sun on snow.
I open my eyes
and see rainbows.

My mother died in mid-December, two weeks after her 97th birthday. On the day of her birthday, we had a small gathering of friends at our home. Outside, it was snowing. I remember my mother, with her silver hair shining, sitting in the center of the circle of guests in her rose-colored satin dressing gown. I remember the magenta petals of the potted cyclamen glowing in the candlelight and the vase of white tea roses on the table. I remember the tiny golden bubbles rising in the champagne flutes, the yellow flames of the fire in the black cast-iron wood stove. I remember vividly the colors of that late afternoon in December, two weeks before her death.

By mid-February, the colors were gone and the whole world looked gray. I had been crying on and off for weeks. My eyes were blinded and swollen, and I was wiped out in the aftermath of her passing. My Heart was weighted down with grief, my head hurt and I had developed a severe sinus infection that would not quit. I had tried various herbal formulas, steams and washes but nothing helped. Finally, a gifted acupuncturist friend offered a treatment.

It had been a long time since I had experienced Bladder 1 - Eyes Bright - *Jing Ming* 睛明. As the needle entered the tiny dip between the two thread-like veins above the medial canthus of my eye, a feeling of relief surged through my body. I knew without a doubt that this point was the doorway to my healing. When the needle reached the qi and paused, I felt a dam of sorrow break as the streams and rivers of my body began to flow once again. My friend withdrew the needle, stood back and wisely waited silently. As I lay on the table, I felt my cheeks flush with warmth and life. My hands and feet tingled with qi and for the first time in many months, there was a faint stirring of joy in my Heart. When I turned my head and looked out the window, I saw the infinite cerulean blue of the sky and I knew that the clear light was returning.

Eyes Bright - *Jing Ming* is a powerful opening point. It is the entryway to the longest meridian in the body and the point where the Bladder, Small Intestine, Stomach, Gall Bladder and Triple Heater meet the Governing Vessel. In modern traditional Chinese medicine, it is recognized as a local point of choice for "virtually any eye disease of external origin...and for the treatment of eye diseases due to interior disharmony, whatever the pathology."[11] For me, it was the doorway back to life.

In naming this point, the ancient physicians intentionally chose the compound character *jing* 睛 rather than the more common simple character *mu* 目 to indicate the eye. While *mu* 目 is an abstracted picture of an actual eye turned sideways, *jing* 睛 places the *mu* radical next to *qing* 青, which combines *sheng* 生, a picture of a sprouting green plant indicating vitality and life, above *dan* 月, a picture of an alchemical furnace indicating both the color red and the alchemical mineral mercuric-sulfide or cinnabar. We find *dan* 月 also used in esoteric language to indicate a process of alchemical transformation. The two radicals taken together in the character *qing* 青 point to the colors produced by processes of transformation in the natural world. *Qing* 青 can refer to green, blue, greenish-black and even cinnabar red, specifically the colors of life rising back at the closing of winter, as well as the potent vitality of birth, youth, growth and rebirth that these colors indicate.

The eye that the point name refers to is not the ordinary eye of the physical body but the portal of spiritual vision, the eye of the enlivening, animating soul of life. In the words of acupuncturist, poet and author Debra Kaatz, "It is where our vision is transformed like the growing insights that come with the alchemist's work of transforming stone into golden elixir."[12]

Furthermore, as Kaatz mentions in her description of this point,[13] *jing* 睛 does not refer to the anatomical eye as a whole but rather to the shining darkness of the eyeball and, specifically, the reflective shimmering blackness of the pupil itself. This reflective blackness of the pupil is related to a fundamental alchemical principle: that the yang light we see in the world around us rises from a ground of yin darkness. Egyptian alchemists referred to this shining fertile blackness as *kem*, the root of our modern word "alchemy." *Kem* refers to the rich, black earth and the fertility of the dark soil of the

Nile valley. In addition, *kem* suggests the black color of lead and other metal ores hidden underground.

But *kem* also had another more esoteric meaning for the Egyptians. The word was used to refer to the shining blackness of the pupil at the center of the eye. The *kem* of the pupil contains a special kind of blackness that is associated not only with its capacity to absorb and transform light into images but also with its ability to act as a tiny mirror that reflects back in miniature the images of the outer world. This reflective capacity of the pupil is especially activated in the presence of the lover who gazes into the eye of the beloved.[14]

When we choose to needle Eyes Bright - *Jing Ming* on a spirit level, we are choosing to ignite the spark of the Fire that illuminates the soul. We are reopening the portals of vision, of a human being's innate capacity to see the colors of the spirit shining back at them from the natural world. Potentially, we are activating a powerful alchemy, a process of transformation that has the potential to renew not only a person's sight but their entire being. In my case, this point revived my soul and brought my spirit back to life. It allowed me to look up to the sky and once again see *ming* 明, the bright, clear light of Heaven illuminating the world. Ultimately, this point helped me to come to a new clarity about death. As I reconnected to my own life force, I came to understand that death can be both a new beginning and an end.

Suggested Needle Technique: Being with Water

It takes great sensitivity, skill, practice and courage on the part of the practitioner to needle this powerful point effectively. And it takes trust and courage on the part of our patients to be willing to receive its gifts. When we call on Eyes Bright - *Jing Ming*, we are calling on the deepest virtues and wisdom of the Water Element. Always discuss and ask the consent of your patient before working with this point. With strong, clear intention, your tiniest needle and your most shallow but most precise insertion will send qi traveling for miles through the waterways of the entire body. Do not be afraid to gently move the eyeball to the side with the fingers of the non-needling hand. And imagine you are going in to ignite the spark of the infinitesimal scintilla, the light seed of the *shen*, the pilot light of the spirit, tucked inside the corner of the eye.

Before needling, pause. Rest in silence. Feel the soles of your feet opening to the streaming life force rising up from below. Remember to ask if the point is available. If the answer is "Yes," take a breath. Then dive!

Bladder 47 (or 52) - Ambition Room - *Zhi Shi*
志室

I wake to winter geese
flying under a full moon.
Wings wide, my spirit rises.

As if in a dream, I walk out into the night and look up to watch as a V of geese passes over my head. Hoarse calls echoing against the cold edges of the night, the birds fly southward, following the courses of the stars. It is late in the season for them to begin their travels, but the unusually warm November weather delayed their departure. Now, they are off! And with powerful wing beats, they race against the coming ice and snow in search of safe haven, food, water and rest.

It takes reserves, resilience, driving instinct, crazy faith and hard-earned wisdom for the geese to make their yearly migration. It takes these same qualities for any being to survive the strenuous demands of winter and the challenges and traumas intrinsic to embodiment: birth, growth, aging and death, betrayal and loss. When a person is overwhelmed by difficulties—floundering in the cold like a downed bird or pushing so hard they have exhausted their resources—opening the door to the Ambition Room can help restore their life force.

I consider Bladder 47 (or 52) - Ambition Room - *Zhi Ji* 志室 when I want to support the foundation of a person's will to live, augment their resiliency and spark their instinctual survival drive. In my practice, I have come across a number of causes for a weak or eroding foundation.

The foundation may be weak due to a variety of prenatal and uterine issues that result in an insufficiency of essences. Prenatal etiologies include inherited ancestral depletion due to multigenerational addiction or malnutrition, genetic mutations due to pharmacological toxicity, extreme hormonal interventions used to induce ovulation and implantation, maternal depression and malnutrition during pregnancy. Postnatal causes include extreme over-exhaustion due to illness and long-term stress, adrenal burnout due to intensive over-work and excess pushing of the will without regard for the physical body's needs.

Another often overlooked cause for a deteriorating foundation is trauma. In this case, the link to source, to lineage and authentic nature, is severed. Water's nourishing connection to ancestral memory is weakened by the amnesia of dissociation and the free and easy flow of the life force rigidifies as the nervous system attempts to block overwhelming emotions including fear and rage.

In all these cases, I have found that Ambition Room - *Zhi Shi* is an important point to consider. As I needle and warm the point, I feel the doors of the Governing Vessel, the Gate of Life, open as well. Vital essences flow from the source to nourish the seed. As the Ambition Room - *Zhi Shi* fills with qi, vitality, stability and integrity return to the foundation. A person may rediscover the reserves, resilience, driving instinct, crazy faith and hard-earned wisdom they need for the life-long journey of return to original nature.

The Chinese point name contains the character *shi* 室, which we will discover again later, embedded in the point name of Bladder 67 - Extremity of Yin - *Zhi Yin*. *Shi* 室 combines the radical 宀 roof with the phonetic *zhi* 至, which sinologist Cecilia Lindqvist describes as "an arrow that has successfully reached its target,"[15] and acupuncturist and scholar Debra Kaatz describes as a picture of "a bird that bends its wings and darts straight down toward the earth."[16] Both interpretations of the character's etymology imply a covered place, a room, where a powerful current of sky qi is directed downward. What rises up from this descent is *zhi* 志, the potent, intrepid and irrepressible sprouting of the will.

Suggested Essential Oil: Cedar

Cedar essential oil is made from one of the largest and longest-living plant organisms on Earth. One look at an Atlas cedar and we understand the nature of will—the *zhi*—the spirit of Water that rises with fierce fortitude and directionality from the dark ground toward the sky. Cedar essential oil endows the spirit with the qualities of endurance, faith and longevity. Herbalist, aromatherapist and author Gabriel Mojay notes that "in contrast to ginger, it does not stimulate the will-power *to action* so much as give us the will *to hold firm*, even against persistent external forces."[17] I turn to this oil when I want to tonify Kidney yang, relieve fatigue, sharpen focus and fortify the will. In addition, it can be used for its gentle, slow, deep and long-lasting stimulating effect on the adrenals.

But the deepest spirit-level action of this oil lies in the tree's ability to endure through time. Not only is the tree itself so long-lived as to be nearly immortal, but the wood is known to resist decay and have potent preserving properties due to the high content of antifungal and antimicrobial factors in its oil. For this reason, I consider cedar essential oil to be a linking agent that can help a person reweave the threads of their lineage to the past as well as to the future. Its rich enlivening fragrance has the capacity to awaken the seed of destiny hidden in Ambition's Room and align the arrow of fate as it rises back toward Heaven from the underworld.

Bladder 58 - Fly and Scatter - *Fei Yang*
飛揚

Big winds after cold rain.
Black branches tear sky holes
in the rushing clouds.

There are winter days when the frozen stillness of the world begins to thaw. It may come early or later in the season, but the thaw is always premature. On these kinds of days, the Green Dragon still sleeps in his bed deep below ground, and the shadow of the black Two-Headed Deer can still be seen, searching for *ling zhi* and gnawing bud-less twigs in the groves. The earth below is sodden, heavy and dark but the sky above is filled with racing clouds. Rain interspersed with driving sleet slants sideways and black crows careen through the trees like tattered bits of crepe paper blowing this way and that in the wind.

This kind of weather is reflected in a patient who is calling out for Bladder 58 - Fly and Scatter - *Fei Yang* 飛揚. Whether due to Water-related fear, anxiety, shock or exhaustion, their thoughts are scattered like those careening crows. Balance on physical, emotional and spiritual levels is disturbed. There is a lack of focus, a tendency toward inexplicable accidents. The line of connection to ground and root has come undone.

This kind of weather can be seen as a split between Heaven and Earth, between the upper and lower extremes of the Bladder meridian. I call on this point for windy, yang signs above or sodden, heavy yin signs below: dizziness in the head or numbness in the toes, cramping tightness in the neck or atrophy in the legs, nasal congestion and nosebleeds or swollen hemorrhoids, a trembling hand and a weak, in-turning ankle.

In addition, since Fly and Scatter - *Fei Yang* is the junction point between the Kidneys and Bladder, it has the unique ability to restore the relationship between the Bladder's righteous stabilizing and storing capacities and the Kidney's receptive filtering and dispersing capacities. I consider it when I suspect a breach in communication between these two officials. Just as freezing rain remains unabsorbed by sodden earth or a wild wind scatters leaves, seeds, feathers and twigs across an unreceptive, infertile ground, the yang Bladder's capacity to control and store may be disconnected from the yin Kidney's capacity to receive, filter and disperse. As these officials come back into communication, their proper functioning is restored. A patient who has been feeling dry, drained and toxic may benefit from this point's particular medicine, as might a patient feeling cold and bloated with fluids.

On a spirit level, the wisdom of this point is embedded in the two characters that make up the point name *Fei Yang* 飛揚. The first character *fei* 飛 contains the radical and phonetic 飞, which pictures a flying crane seen from the side. This graphic expresses the simplicity, ease and grace of the bird's flight, the delicate head with long neck extended forward and the tail extended back with the two wings fluttering at the side. The second character *yang* 揚 means to raise or spread. *Yang* contains the radical *shou* 手 hand, which means grasp or have in hand. Through these embedded symbols, I understand that Fly and Scatter - *Fei Yang* has the power to restore grace and flow to the Water Element so that blood, fluids, thoughts and emotions can all move freely like the white crane who flies with smooth, rhythmic wingbeats over the dark marsh. And, like a skillful hand gentling a panicking wild creature, this same point can gather up and grasp untethered, scattered qi so that the receptive, quiescent, gestational potency of the Water Element can be restored until it is truly time for the winds of Spring to wake the sleeping dragon.

Suggested Needle Technique: Grasping the Qi

In working with this point, I find that it is important for the needle to strongly grasp the qi and for the patient to feel a sensation that extends away from the point and down the leg, often with a scattering of *de qi* down into the foot, in order to activate its full effect. I needle in the direction of the flow of the meridian and check in with the patient to make sure there is significant sensation before withdrawing the needle. If the symptoms include accumulation, deficiency or blockage in the lower body, I often burn a moxa cone directly on the needle to further amplify the activating, yang aspect of the treatment.

Bladder 60 - Kunlun Mountain - *Kunlun*
崑崙

At winter's still point
alone in the night, I stand
with the turning stars.

For Taoists, Kunlun Mountain is the mythical center pole of the universe. In the cosmos, it is the *axis mundi*, the pillar that stands between Heaven and Earth, Above and Below. In the body, it is the spinal column, the vertical axis of our being. I have written previously, "The mountain is...the connecting link between our body, our spirit, our mind and our soul. The labyrinths below the mountain represent the primal, instinctual wisdom of our bodies while the North Star, which shines at the mountaintop, represents the speck of spirit whose light guides our journey from birth through life and back to our original nature."[18] The Mountain symbolizes the stabilized wholeness of the self, our capacity for reflective, restful tranquility and determined, effective movement when the time is right. In the words of the *I Ching*, "a mountain is at peace with itself and there is nothing stronger or more mighty."[19]

Bladder 60 - Kunlun Mountain - *Kunlun* 崑崙, like the mountain it is named for, is the great stabilizer. It has the paradoxical capacity to descend, center and ground but also to activate and move. Its descending effect can be felt along the entire length of the Bladder channel. Indeed, as the *I Ching* implies, through its ability to clear heat and wind in the channel and lead excess heat and yang qi downward, the Mountain brings peace to the spirit and easeful balance to the body.

Yet, as the Fire point on the Bladder meridian, Kunlun Mountain - *Kunlun* can also be used to warm frozen Water or help to reignite the yang spark of life in the Kidneys after adrenal burnout. By engaging the yang energy of the Fire within, Kunlun Mountain - *Kunlun* helps to release physical or emotional contraction and counteract states of fearful withdrawal. It restores movement and flow when a lack of yang qi has resulted in the stagnation of fluids and, in this way, it can help to reverse symptoms such as edema, boggy lethargy and lack of drive. The point has a beneficial effect of bringing warmth and suppleness to the physical spine, and it also supports the backbone in a psychological sense, bringing strength, conviction and centering as its gifts.

In the poem "The Ode to the Jade Dragon," attributed to the 12th-century Taoist sage and acupuncturist Ma Danyang,[20] Kunlun Mountain - *Kunlun* is included on the list as one of the Twelve Heavenly Star Points. Danyang considered these 12 points to be crucial to the practice of acupuncture, perhaps even the only points an acupuncturist needs in order to become a master of the craft. In the poem, he wrote, "All 360 holes do not escape these 12 strange charms, healing a disease is like magic... A torrent whirling as wind-driven snow, the Northern Dipper sends down its true workings."[21]

Danyang's indications for the use of Kunlun Mountain - *Kunlun* reinforce our understanding of the point's paradoxical effects. According to Danyang's ode, the point relieves spasms and pain in the tailbone due to injury resulting in stagnation and excess. It relieves fullness in the chest that results in shortness of breath. On the deficiency side, it can be called on when a person can raise their leg and yet feels "unable to walk, or even step out."[22] Danyang also says to consider the point when "you move just once and immediately groan."[23] For me, this final entry speaks of the point's profound effect on the spirit of Water. It reinvigorates the *zhi*, thus restoring a person's will to move, explore and engage with life. Last but not least, tapping the magic of this mythical mountain alleviates excessive groaning and brings a lilting note of joy back to the Water's music.

Suggested Essential Oil: Nutmeg

Nutmeg is an evergreen shrub that thrives in humid climates. It dislikes direct heat and sunlight, does best in moist, well-drained soil and has a particular affinity for the forest understory at the lower altitudes of hillsides and mountains. The warming nature of the oil reminds me of the embers of coal that persist after the initial flames of a fire have burned down. Nutmeg essential oil tonifies Kidney yang and I have found it to be useful for adrenal insufficiency, lack of energy, lack of ambition, nervous fears and low libido.

During ancient times, Roman and Greek civilizations used nutmeg as a brain tonic. More recent research has shown that it has neuroprotective properties.[24] Additionally, nutmeg's volatile oils have been shown to increase the levels of serotonin, dopamine and norepinephrine in the hippocampus, which is the part of the brain responsible for memory and spatial navigation. In addition, I find that it has a brightening yet calming effect on the mind. When I apply a drop of this oil to Kunlun Mountain - *Kunlun*, I am following the well-known traditional Chinese medicine principle that states, "for diseases of the head select points from the feet."[255] As I work at the base of the mountain, I can resolve problems on the mountain top and encourage the qi to flow harmoniously through the body.

Nutmeg essential oil is strong and the aroma is somewhat cloying. It should be used judiciously, diluted or in very small amounts but, when indicated, will bring a warming, enlivening effect to all aspects of the inner mountain.

Bladder 67 - Extremity of Yin - *Zhi Yin*
至陰

*Sparrows puff their feathers
in the cold wind, as each day,
the sun grows stronger.*

Sometimes it is hard to know when gestation is complete. When is it dark enough? Quiet enough? When have I had enough rest, sufficient time to prepare for the journey ahead? When have I stored adequate resources? When is it time to turn?

This is the question that the soul of the seed asks before sprouting in the darkness. It is the question that the baby in the womb asks during the last weeks of pregnancy. And it is the question we all ask at pivotal transformational moments in our lives.

We find a clue to the answer to this question in the spirit of the point, Bladder 67 - Extremity of Yin - *Zhi Yin* 至陰. The Bladder channel descends from the inner canthus of the eyes, over the head and down the spine and the back of the legs until it reaches the lowest point, the tip of the little toe. It arrives at the turning point, Extremity of Yin - *Zhi Yin*, the extreme expression of yin on the Bladder channel. Here, the qi reverses back along the sole of the foot to rise again through Kidney 1 - Bubbling Spring - *Yong Guan* and shoots upward through the Kidney and *Chong Mai* channels. The energies of descent, darkness, rest and gestation transform into the energies of ascension, light, activation and birth.

The character *zhi* 至 is derived from an ancient graphic that pictures an arrow heading downward to the horizon line of the Earth, described by sinologist Cecilia Lindqvist as "an arrow that has successfully reached its target."[266] In an alternative interpretation, Debra Kaatz describes the character as a picture of "a bird that bends its wings and darts straight down toward the earth."[277]

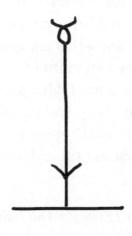

ZHI - WILL

Zhi 至 is translated as "to reach, to arrive at, until" and in Extremity of Yin - *Zhi Yin* it implies that we have arrived at the most extreme point; we have hit the target. The word is a homonym for the spirit of Water, the *zhi* 志 ambition or will of the Kidneys. It is also worth noting that there is an echoing in *zhi* 至 of the graphic *shi* 士, a sprouting plant emerging from the soil and a yang phallic symbol that we find rising from *xin* 心 the Heart in *zhi* 志.

I have a great depth of gratitude for the powerfully awakening and activating seed of yang that is planted in darkness at Extremity of Yin - *Zhi Yin*. This seed has opened its medicine in my treatment room in many miraculous ways. More than once, I have been asked to intervene when a Cesarean section is looming on the horizon for a mother whose baby persists in a cozy transverse position even after the time has come to turn. It is an awe-inspiring thing when, after many, many applications of rice grain moxa, after chanting, singing and dancing over this point, I perceive the first quickening: a harmonizing pulse, a deepening breath, a brightening in the complexion. Later in the night, I see my phone light up with the text: "It happened. There was a lot of movement in the belly and now we can feel it! The head is down." Then I know that the arrow hit the mark! The treatment reached the extremity of yin and the yang seed sprouted. The little bird has folded its wings and is darting toward the Earth. The baby has turned head down and is ready to enter the birth canal, prepared for the next waves of change, waiting to descend through the darkness, to rise to meet the light.

Suggested Essential Oil: Balsam Fir

The exudation of this tree is a sticky brownish-golden sap. The sap has long been recognized for its medicinal uses and the tree itself is named for it. The word "balsam" is used in alchemy to refer to a substance—a balm—that has deep, even sacred, healing properties.

I reach for balsam fir essential oil when the Water Element has reached the depth of its darkness and it is time to bring in the light. Like the solstice season that this tree is so often associated with, the scent of balsam opens my heart to the feeling of faith that is a hallmark of a healthy Water Element. I call on this calming, rooting and at the same time wildly invigorating fragrance when I want to honor the softness and wisdom of the yin as well as the energizing spark of the yang within it.

Kidney 1 - Bubbling Spring - *Yong Guan*
涌泉

Gush of light, this ice
so full of life awakens.
I drink deep and walk on.

I remember with crystal clarity the first time, more than 30 years ago, that I experienced the transformative nature of Kidney 1 - Bubbling Spring - *Yong Guan* 涌泉. I arrived for my acupuncture session in a state of fiery hyperactivity, nearly manic with an exuberance of anxiety and chatter. Although I can no longer remember the outer events that precipitated my heightened emotional state, I remember the feeling of agitation and inner turmoil, the thoughts spinning wildly through my brain. My acupuncturist took one look at me and told me to take off my socks and go lie down on the treatment table.

I was alarmed when I realized that she was looking for a point on the bottom of my foot but before I had time to question her decision, she said, "Take a breath." As the needle entered the powerful stream of the Kidney meridian, I felt my spirit land back in my body. I was calm, relaxed and present, as if I had been dipped in a pool of tranquility. What I learned that day is that when this point is needled when necessary, there is no pain, only a sense of relief and the profound pleasure of being met, touched and rooted deeply back in one's own being.

The character *yong* 涌 combines an abbreviation of the Water radical *shui* 氵 with the radical *yong* 甬. The phonetic *yong* 用 is a picture of a target pierced through the center by an arrow. The little triangular mark on top of *yong* 甬 represents an emerging sprout of grass or a blooming flower. The energy is direct, upward-moving, vibrant. It depicts a vital force that bursts forth directly from its source. The accompanying character *quan* combines the full radical *shui* 水 beneath *bai* 白, meaning white or bright, pictured as the sun with a ray of light rising above it. *Quan* reinforces the idea of clear yang light rising up from dark yin Water. The two characters together graphically depict water gushing or bubbling up from an underground spring.

The name *Yong Quan* 涌泉 tells us that this is the point where the downward yin tendency of Water reverses and gushes upward, clear and pure, from the dark recesses of the Earth. As the Wood point of the Water, Bubbling Spring - *Yong Guan* combines the directedness and hopefulness of Spring with the gestational power and resourcefulness of Winter. It is the deep-down place where the secret potency of the green sprout is stored.

We go to this spring when we need to replenish our souls and rejuvenate our bodies. We go down to find the negentropic upward thrust of the life force of the Earth. It is no accident that a body-felt sense connection to Bubbling Spring - *Yong Guan* is considered the foundation of skillful *qi gong* and yoga practice and that any movement upwards in *tai qi* begins by rooting down into the earth through this point at the bottom of the feet.

Needling this point calms the spirit and energizes and replenishes the essences. The point has a grounding and rooting effect, yet it also has the capacity to lift and lighten the qi. It is indicated when there is a need to restrain uprising heat, for states of agitation, insomnia and fear and even rage and madness with "a desire to kill people."[288] And yet, as the entry and *jing*-well, it can also be called on when there is a need to lift, revive, restore and energize the qi and reverse collapsing yang. Due to its adaptogenic nature, Bubbling Spring - *Yong Guan* offers relief in cases where rising yin deficiency heat alternates with cold, such as menopausal hot flashes and night sweats.

Suggested Treatment Strategy: Moxa Pole

Over the years, I have come to respect the power of this point and its extreme sensitivity to stimulus. In general, I use a relatively slim needle and am judicious about depth, only inserting to the place where I feel the qi begin to stir. I also use acupressure, essential oils, direct rice grain moxa and tuning forks with very good effect.

One of my favorite ways to tap the wisdom of Bubbling Spring - *Yong Guan* is with a moxa pole. In this case, I hold the pole about an inch away from the foot and draw slow, steady circles around the point. One of the most amazing and immediate changes I see when gently warming the point in this way is with emotional upset due to counterflow qi in the *Chong Mai*, when gracious communication between the Kidneys and Heart is impeded or blocked. I offer this treatment when a patient comes in complaining of anxiety, trembling agitation, Running Piglet Syndrome, through the upper *dan tian* and throat. I continue the circling of the pole until the breath becomes rhythmic and smooth, the muscles relax, color returns to the face and steady light returns to the eyes. Then I pause and remember my own first experience of drinking the waters of this spring, and I am filled with gratitude for the mysterious power of our medicine.

Kidney 3 - Greater Mountain Stream - *Tai Xi*
太谿

Morning after rain,
last leaves glow golden in the ice
blue thunder of the sky.

Winter days are brief and often spare in their offerings. On these days, the world is heavy and contracted. The frozen ground whispers, "Wait...wait...wait."

But on this morning, after a wild night of rain, the temperature rises just a degree or two above freezing. A skittering wind darts between the tree branches and brushes the cobwebs of clouds from the sky. There is a liveliness to the light: diamond-bright yet freely flowing directly down from the blue sea of Heaven. A day like this speaks not only to the restorative, preserving and gestational potency of the Water Element but also to the invigorating and rejuvenating qualities of the cold and the spontaneous delight, playfulness and creativity that is part of Water's intrinsic nature. When I want to access this aspect of Water's medicine, I go to Kidney 3 - Greater Mountain Stream - *Tai Xi* 太谿.

The great wisdom of this point is that it goes down to go up. When I want to tap its tonifying, enlivening properties, I go to the place where the meridian temporarily reverses. I angle the needle down toward the bottom of the foot, in the direction of flow toward Kidney 5 - Water Spring - *Shui Quan* and Kidney 6 - Shining Sea - *Zhao Hai*. I go down toward the yin in order to tap the qi at the source. If I follow the stream far enough, I discover that it returns at Kidney 7 - Returning Current - *Fu Liu* and rises from the darkness through Kidney 21 - Hidden Gate - *You Men* to illuminate the Kidney points of the upper mansion of the chest.

As the *Yuan* source point on the Kidney meridian, the point is adaptogenic. It descends to the wellspring of the qi and brings back what is needed. For depletion and exhaustion, it brings replenishing nourishment, strength and endurance. When there is shakiness, agitation and excess emotion, it brings peace and calm. It nourishes yin, clears heat and treats disharmony at every level of the Water Element.

As the Earth point on the Kidney meridian, it carries the Earth's legacy of stability and sweetness across the K'o cycle to its grandchild. Through this point, the Earth gifts its grandchild with nourishment, containment, harmony and endurance. I call on this aspect of Greater Mountain Stream - *Tai Xi* when a patient's Water is weak, flowing irregularly or without control, particularly when the Earth qi is strong and the Kidney qi weak. Consider this possibility when there are symptoms such as enuresis, frequent, copious urination, cold limbs, shakiness, anxiety and a lack of a feeling of grounding and center.

The name emphasizes the importance of this point by using the character *tai* 太 greater, rather than *tai* 大 great. Here, the picture of a grown person with arms and legs outstretched 大 has an added stroke 太 to reinforce the supreme, extraordinary, fully expressed power of the greatness. The accompanying character *xi* 谿 is a picture of a weaver 奚—a person beneath the radical for silk threads—and *gu* 谷 a picture of the *kou* 口 mouth of a gorge or valley. The character reinforces our sense of this point as the great disseminator, the one who works the threads—the rivulets, brooks and streams—of the Water so that they weave through every aspect of our being. From the Greater Mountain Stream, Water flows from the source, rising up from the ground in a gushing torrent of life force that quenches, nourishes and awakens us at the level of body, soul and spirit.

Suggested Essential Oil: Sweet Birch Bark

Birch trees flourish in northern climates. They thrive in cool, moist soil and their shallow roots make them sensitive to heat or drought. Birch is a thirsty tree that soaks up copious amounts of moisture from the ground. Thus, the oil derived from the bark of this tree has a strong affinity with the Water Element as well as the Earth. It has the capacity to support the Bladder with the appropriate control and storage of fluids and the Kidneys with filtration and detoxification.

On a physical level, this oil can be used as an adjunct to other treatments. It can help promote the flow of urine, reduce edema, lower high blood pressure and reduce the severity of urinary tract infections. A drop of the neat oil applied directly to the point can be combined with a gentle abdominal massage using a few drops of birch bark essential oil well blended in a carrier oil.

On the level of the spirit, the oil has a cooling, calming and at the same time brightening effect. Imagine western light drifting through the branches in a sunlit birch grove on a winter afternoon and you get a sense of its alchemical potency: its sweet but resilient nature, its quiet yet determined presence, its clarity and peaceful atmosphere. The oil has a spare yet generous wintry aroma that activates and spreads the crystalline clarity and quiet thunder of Greater Mountain Stream - *Tai Xi*.

Kidney 7 - Returning Current - *Fu Liu*
復溜

Deep below the melting snow
some green memory wakens
and life rushes upward.

After a time of decay comes the turning point. The
powerful light that has been banished returns. There is
movement but it is not brought about by force.

I Ching: Hexagram 24 - Return - *Fu*[299]

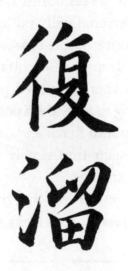

At the still point of winter, a black line cracks the ice. January thaws and, deep below the Earth, seeds stir and turn in their underworld beds. Now is the season of Water. Water's medicine is gestation, the capacity of the yin to carry an embryo, seed or new possibility safely sequestered within a womb-like vessel until it is ready to emerge from darkness into light.

Water is yin but it is also the birthplace of the yang. This *enantiodromia*—the spontaneous emergence of the opposite when some quality or stage reaches its fullest expression— is a governing principle of natural cycles and psychological development. It is also one of the great mysteries of the Water Element. The emergence of the yang from the yin that occurs in the Water is the blue spark that reignites the engine of the life cycle as we move through Winter back to Spring. It is the vital force that reanimates the soul, the impossible miracle of resurrection after devastation that is hidden at the heart of the alchemical quest.

Water tells us that this renewal is possible but it can only come through a descent into darkness. It cannot be forced through the personal will and its timing is not under conscious control. Winter is the season of faith. It is a time to reach down to the deepest reservoirs of our being, to trust that in this darkness there is a seed preparing to sprout, a hidden vitality waiting to activate, a potency that transforms will into wisdom, fear into fierce and dedicated courage, and not knowing and despair into timely, skillful and effective action in the coming spring.

The mysterious *enantiodromia* that happens at the turning point of Water is expressed in *Fu* Hexagram 24 of the *I Ching*.

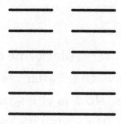

HEXAGRAM 24 - RETURN - *FU*

The unbroken yang line beneath the five broken yin lines represents the awakening of the seed and the rebirth of yang potency, activity and growth from deep in the yin darkness. It represents the beginning of a new cycle. This hexagram is associated with the month of January, the weeks after the winter solstice when the days grow longer and the light returns.

Kidney 7 - Returning Current - *Fu Liu* 復溜 carries the medicine of this potent returning aspect of the Water. When we open this point, it is as if we have cleared away a blockage in a stream. Without force or effort, the current once again begins to flow. This Water point brings vitality back to our being. On the spirit level, it is a point of rebirth. It restores our faith in our own resiliency and reawakens our desires, drives and will to live.

Returning Current - *Fu Liu* is the turning point. The point is located on the Kidney meridian where the current of the qi that has reversed downwards at Kidney 3 - Greater Mountain Stream - *Tai Xi* turns back up toward the yang, the torso and the light. As the Metal in the Water of the Kidney meridian, this point has the power to pull the qi back from the right yin to the left, yang side of the *sheng* or life cycle of the Five Elements.

Consider this point when a person is disheartened, is exhausted or has completely lost touch with the river of their Tao. Consider it when there is a need for someone or something to be reborn. Consider it when action proceeds without the stabilizing influence of wisdom and when the light of faith no longer illuminates the darkness of the world.

Through this point, the yin's tendency toward entropy is reversed. We can once again dare to stand against the forces of disintegration and death. The streams, rivers and oceans of life begin to flow again. As we read in Hexagram 24 of the

I Ching, "The transformation of the old becomes easy. The old is discarded and the new is introduced."[30]

Suggested Essential Oil: Juniper

Juniper essential oil is a primary oil for the Water Element. The English name "juniper" is derived from the Latin *juniores*, which means "young berries," and the name attunes us to the plant's capacity to rejuvenate and reverse the effects of aging, also a part of the Water Element's medicine. The blue berries stay fresh at the tips of the evergreen branches through the winter and are another reminder of the plant's tenacity and resilience. Juniper warms and stimulates Kidney yang. In the process, it strengthens the will and our capacity to stand strong and upright in the face of adversity. It drives out negativity and relieves the fear of failure. Applied to Kidney 7 - Returning Current - *Fu Liu*, this oil activates the forces of life and brings vitality back to the soul.

Kidney 16 - Vitals Transfer Point - *Huang Shu*

肓俞

Last night, the waning moon
sailed through my dreams; this morning
seafoam frosts my windows.

Here is the first image I have of my granddaughter: she is just born, her face a bit bruised from her long, night-sea journey through the birth canal. Her back is rounded and her little legs are drawn into her chest as her body instinctively returns to its familiar fetal curl. Her eyes are dazed by the dim light but open, aware. And from the center of her belly, she is still connected for these last few moments to her mother by a powerful, crimson cord of flesh throbbing with blood, qi and nutrients for her body, her soul and her spirit.

As the cord is cut, I watch as her *po* soul rises from her belly to her Lungs and she takes her first breath. She flings her arms wide, opens her tiny mouth and gives a wail of greeting to the world. Then, back on her mother's body, she begins to take in nourishment in a whole new way.

Each one of us has gone through this process. Each of us in our own way leaves behind the floating world of the womb and the effortless flow of nutrients delivered directly to the center of our being. Each of us has had to discover over time how to nourish ourselves differently. Yet the memory of that umbilical connection remains in the recesses of our cellular memory: the belly as the place where we once received the miraculous materials that brought us into being. When I feel a patient needs to remember this time of yin connection to the source, I turn to Kidney 16 - Vitals Transfer Point - *Huang Shu* 肓俞.

Of all the points I work with in the body, Kidney 16 - Vitals Transfer Point - *Huang Shu* is the one that patients express the most gratitude for. Inevitably, as I insert the needle, apply warmth with stick moxa or a heat lamp, massage the area with qi-moving oils or activate the blood with gentle *qua sha*, there is a sigh of relaxation and relief generally followed by words like, "That heat is just what I needed," "I feel qi moving down into my legs," or "That feels so good." I think of this point as the gateway to the "mother." When I choose to use it, which is often, particularly during the colder months of the year, I hold the intention of opening a person to the ocean of qi that once effortlessly nourished them, the ocean that that still swirls in the deepest part of our bodies: the lower *dan tian*.

Vitals Transfer Point - *Huang Shu*, located on either side of the umbilicus, is a point that brings us back to our origin, to the body-felt sense memory of the womb where we gestated in a timeless, spaceless dream. It brings us back to a place of rest where the body can be revitalized and the spirit calmed until the yang seed is ready to sprout from the yin and it is time to emerge from darkness into light.

I have used the point with great success to relieve abdominal tightness, particularly with cold signs, menstrual discomfort and exhaustion, and also for states of anxiety related to disharmony in the central channel of the *Chong Mai* meridian that passes directly through this point. I find that touching Vitals Transfer Point - *Huang Shu* has the almost immediate effect of shifting agitation to relaxation and encouraging constrained qi to flow harmoniously.

The idea that this point activates a direct transfer of qi to the deepest, most crucial parts of our being is expressed in the point name. *Huang* combines the radical *rou* 月 meaning flesh with *wang* 亡 which is a picture of a nook or hiding place. It can also be seen as a grave or a place of burial. That radical 亡 is used to mean die. The two radicals taken together 肓 imply a hidden, tucked-away part of our physical body, a hiding place for flesh without which we would die; in other words, the vital organs that are tucked away, hidden in the belly.

The character *shu* 俞 contains the radical *you* 月. This radical is used in *huang* to mean *rou* flesh. In the second radical, the same radical is said to be a small boat, pictured going upstream toward a delta, a triangular shape that archetypally has always been a shorthand sign for the female pelvis. The character *you* 月 is also most commonly used to mean moon.

So here in the point name we discover the inner meaning, the spirit of this point: Vitals Transfer Point - *Huang Shu* is the docking place where the moon boat of the yin waits with its bounty of shining essences and vitalizing qi. When we tap this point, we release the little boat from its mooring and send it down to the deep waters of the *dan tian* where it delivers its precious cargo of warmth, blood, qi and nutrients to the place where the energies of life originate: our vitals.

Suggested Treatment Strategy: Sending Down the Boat

One caveat when considering Vitals Transfer Point - *Huang Shu* is that it is very important to ask for consent before treatment. The area where this point is located is vulnerable. After all, it is the hiding place of our "vitals" and for some people, especially those with a history of abuse or boundary violation, even gentle touch may feel invasive. Once consent is granted, my experience is that the point responds with gratitude to most forms of gentle warming and tonification. Whatever modality I choose, my intention is to "send the moon boat" to the core of a person's being.

When using needles, I direct them slightly downward toward the pelvis and inward toward the Conception Vessel. The qi can be surprisingly deep here, so I continue to penetrate the flesh with great care and caution until I reach the channel and feel a grab on the needle. Essential oils are another treatment of choice. One favorite is fennel, which has the dual effect of warming and moving qi in the abdomen, aiding digestion and relieving spasms. But my all-time favorite with patients showing any kind of cold signs is stick moxa. I find this gradual and gentle warming is the best way to get the little boat moving along the currents of the meridians, transporting what is needed to the place where we need it most.

Kidney 25 - Spirit Storehouse - *Shen Cang*
神藏

Some flowers blossom
in the snow. Lost treasure found
when least expected.

First snow. Already, it's beginning to melt. The world is wet, sodden and cold. In my treatment room, I find the Lung pulse often buried deep under a thick quilt of silence. Even with needles and grains of fiery moxa, it is hard to ignite the enlivening breath. Outside, in the early afternoon, the light is already sinking behind the clouds, burrowing down early, waking late.

Throughout this autumn, I have followed the threads of the public conversation. Sexual harassment. Refugees. Terrorists. Taxes. #MeToo. Nuclear war. Words torn into scraps fall like ash from the sky and accumulate in useless piles along the sides of my inner landscape. Now, as darkness descends, I want to sweep it all away and find the place where the new clear Water will rise, springing up again from down below. Here is where I will wait this winter to welcome back the light.

The atmosphere of this time is represented by the *I Ching* in Hexagram 36 - The Darkening of the Light - *Ming Yi*. Here we read, "The sun has sunk under the earth and is therefore darkened. The bright is wounded. A man of grievous nature is in a position of authority and brings harm to the wise and able."[311] We have arrived at a time of adversity and yet the oracle tells us: "One must not unresistingly let himself be swept along by unfavorable circumstances, nor permit his steadfastness to be shaken. He can avoid this by maintaining his inner light...in some situations indeed a man must hide his light, in order to make his will prevail in spite of difficulties... perseverance must dwell in inmost consciousness."[322]

Kidney 25 - Spirit Storehouse - *Shen Cang* 神藏 offers healing for this time of adversity when yang light is nearly extinguished in the dark yin depths of winter. The point is found on the upper aspect of the Kidney meridian. It is located in the second intercostal space, two finger widths away from the centerline. It hovers just above the Lungs at the level of the upper edge of the Heart.

The name of the point combines the character *shen* 神 spirit with the character *cang* 藏 meaning to store, conceal or hide. *Cang* implies not only the storing away of what is valuable for later use but also the idea of hibernation, of going inward, of passing through the lean months of winter by dropping into a deep state of rest.

The minister who resides at the center of this point cradles the *shen* like a restless bird safely beneath her silken robes. There, in the dark, the wounded wings of the light can heal.

In current times, our world often seems too painful to bear, but this point reminds us that gradually radiance will return to the Earth. Deep in the storehouse, the seeds wait until it is once again appropriate to grow. This waiting is not the same as doing nothing. Rather, it is like winnowing, separating the precious from the worthless, breathing in what truly inspires us and breathing out what we no longer need. In this way, in a time of darkness, we veil our light and yet continue to shine.

We can touch Spirit Storehouse - *Shen Cang* when:

- on a physical level, a person is experiencing pain and oppression of the chest or having difficulty taking a full breath. This constriction may be due to asthma or lingering coughs but also when there is unfinished grief, a withholding of the breath to avoid the release of sobbing or letting go of someone or something dearly loved.

- Winter and the Water Element call us toward introversion, rest and restoration. When we feel vulnerable or when the outer world assaults or overly distracts us from our own inner knowing, we can call on Spirit Storehouse - *Shen Cang* to offer a place of refuge and relief.

- there is a need to go in deep to restore the soul, to rediscover our stability and power in the face of great loss, disillusionment or betrayal.

- there is some hidden emotion, story or prayer that needs to mature and ripen before being revealed. This point offers the gift of right timing.

- our inner and outer worlds are out of alignment. When we need to attend to what is coming to life within us in order to bring our gifts more skillfully out into the world.

Suggested Treatment Strategy: Less is More

Be sure to use care when needling this point, particularly with thinner, less muscular patients, as the tender organs of the Heart and Lungs lie just beneath. Transverse, oblique needling directed laterally is recommended. I find that gentle needling with finer needles is usually more effective when working at the spirit level, so remember that less is not only safer but very often more effective.

This point responds beautifully to rice grain moxa, particularly when there is sadness, despair, depression or recent loss. Three to five grains is usually sufficient.

Consider cedarwood essential oil to calm, fortify and root the *shen* and to offer endurance during times of crisis and challenge. Cedar provides a sense of deep spiritual certainty and unwavering determination that complements the faith and patience of this point. Together, point and oil support us in transforming a dangerous or disheartening situation into an experience from which we can grow in wisdom, skill and deeply rooted power. In this way, we move beyond temporary hindrances and persevere until the light returns from its seclusion in the darkness.

Wood: Spring Season

Wood pushes upward from the dark Earth, sprouts, grows and goes its own way toward the sky. While its roots sink down to drink the dark mineral-rich waters of the Earth, Wood's leafy branches spread up toward Heaven to transform the Fire of sunlight into food. Wood is the connecting link between Above and Below, Heaven and Earth. It melds the powers of yin and yang into a unique living organism that can move forward into its own future. It may sprout suddenly from bog-like skunk cabbage, grow in a primeval forest with slow, determined power like a sequoia or snake resolutely up a bean pole. But however it goes, it grows! Wood is life becoming! The Wood Element lives in us, not only in the tensile strength of our tendons and ligaments, the clarity of our eyesight, the luster of our fingernails and the fluidity of our tears, but also in our souls.

The Chinese character for Wood is *mu* 木. The character is a picture of a tree, roots reaching down and branches extending out and upward. At the center is the trunk, the vertical axis that balances polarities and allows the energies of life to flow simultaneously in two directions through the tree.

In traditional Chinese medicine, Wood is related to the season of Spring. It represents the time of year when, after winter's long, dark days of yin gathering, storing, compression and gestating, the yang life force activates, expands and re-emerges from the underworld. The Wood Element marks the return of life, the time of year when, in the words of poet Ezra Pound, "every branch has back what last year lost."[1] Wood is the energy of birth, sprouting, healthy aggression, creativity and the fierce desire to take one's place in the dance of life. It is an expression of qi that is warming, directed and determined. Like the season of Spring, Wood is related to birth and growth but also to the blueprint of life— the inherent order, purpose and plan of being—the aspect of Tao that informs the unfolding of living structures.

On the Five Element Wheel, we find Wood on the left yang negentropic side, between the sustaining, rooting support of the yin of Water and the initiating, blossoming uplift of yang Fire. This placement reflects Wood's capacity to resolve the tension of opposites and affirms its tendency to negate entropy, to expand, move toward the light and grow toward states of greater complexity and power. After a time of sleep, the hard seeds soften, the first green shoots poke up from the soil as the power of hope and possibility returns to the cosmos.

Kigo words evoke the atmosphere of fierce exuberance, vitality, freshness and determined hope that is the hallmark of Wood. Yet they also remind us of Wood's other face, the softness, delicacy, tentative vulnerability and the gradually increasing warmth that infuses the spring with its exquisite tenderness and beauty. Waking at night to the croaking of early tree frogs. Leisurely strolling under umbrellas to view the cherry trees blossoming in the April rain. Easy wandering along woodland paths. The warbler serenading his mate. The young ram charging up the hillside. Southerly winds and warm mist obscuring the moon. Shoots of green peas and radish in the garden, nettles, fiddleheads and wild onion in the field. Wood brings us to the immediacy, passion and poignancy of adolescence tempered by the age-old knowledge of the tree of life itself.

Vegetative Expression

The vegetative expression of this Element is the young green sprout that defies the force of gravity as it rises up from the dark ground. The spirit of this Element can be seen in the first blade of shining grass that pushes up through the cold, hard ground of late March—resolute, vigorous, directed. Like that first blade of grass, the Wood Element expresses the quality of vision, hope, future possibilities and redemption. The green sprout is the vegetative archetype of arousal, growth, directionality and the pioneering spirit that are primary functions of this Element. In the words of the second-century Chinese text the *Baihutong*, "The term 'wood' (*mu*) means 'to butt'; the yang qi rouse and butt at the earth to come out."[2]

When the seed germinates in the dark depths of Water, the Wood Element is already planning its ultimate form, function and direction toward the sky.

Color/Sound/Odor/Emotion

The Color of Wood is Green

In the *Neijing Suwen*, we read, "Green is the color of the East, it pervades the Liver and lays open the eyes...its kind is grass and trees."[3] To diagnose the health of the Wood Element, look at the sides of the eyes, temples and laugh lines around the mouth for a range from rich blue-green spruce to newly sprouting leaves. The *Neijing Suwen* also tells us, "When their color is green like grass they are without life... When their color is green like a kingfisher's wing they are full of life."[4] Study green in nature in both balance and imbalance, and notice how your heart responds.

The Sound is Shout

Listen for a voice that either comes at you with strong, clear enunciation (excess Wood) or barely makes its way in a whisper across a room (deficient Wood). This sound of shouting may actually be a markedly loud voice or it may be a normal-range sound level that is characterized by its confidence and demand for attention. Remember that lack of shout can also be the sound of Wood.

The Odor is Rancid

In balance, rancid is like fresh-pressed oil and it tells us that the Liver and Gall Bladder are doing their job of processing nutrients and fats in the body. When out of balance, rancid is like the smell of oil that has been sitting too long in a jar or the last bit of butter in the butter dish. This out-of-balance rancid smell tells us that the body is having difficulty metabolizing both food and life impressions.

The Emotion is Anger

In health, the emotion of Wood expresses as an easy unforced clarity of direction and action, a vitality of imagination and certainty of vision. Out of balance, this can manifest as outright irritability and aggression. It can also show up as timidity and an inability to speak up for one's own individual needs or to make a clear decision about small details or large life plans.

The Officials

Wood is related to the organs of the Liver and Gall Bladder. It has to do with the storage, detoxification and movement of blood, the resilience and vitality of our connective tissue and the health of our eyes. Just as a healthy tree extends its leaves upward to capture its own bit of sunlight and its roots downward to soak up rain, healthy Wood allows us to move with decisiveness toward what we need in order to manifest our true nature. The Wood Element knows where we begin and end! It recognizes our edges and boundaries and allows us to affirm them appropriately.

The yin Liver and yang Gall Bladder function in close relationship to each other. One way to understand the complex relationship between these two officials is to consider the overall shape of a tree as the function of the Liver Official. Even from a distance, we can distinguish the difference between a weeping willow, a spruce tree and a birch. Yet this overall shape is created through an ongoing unfolding of minute twists and turns of trunk, branch, stem, twig and leaf. Each of these twists and turns represents a decision as to how to make the best use of available resources while continuing to express the essential nature of that particular tree. The micro-decisions to go one way or the other at a particular moment in time come under the jurisdiction of the Gall Bladder.

The Liver Official is said to hold the office of General of the Armed Forces. We can also think of the Liver as the architect, the master planner and the designer of the individual self. The Liver initiates the project and leads the way into the creative processes of being. Vision, on physical, psychological and spiritual levels, is key to its function. Symptoms related to the eyes, the blood, sleeping and dreaming along with the flexibility and strength of the tendons and ligaments are all related to this official.

The Gall Bladder Official holds the office of Direction and Decision Making. The Gall Bladder determines the correctness of decisions that are to carry the Liver's plan forward into action. "Choice" is key to the function of the Gall Bladder. When this function is impaired, the master plan and vision of the Liver cannot be put into action. Along with chronic indecisiveness and procrastination, problems with balance and coordination as well as one-sided symptoms are often related to the Gall Bladder.

Hun: The Spirit of Wood

The spirit of Wood is the *hun* 魂, which is translated as ethereal soul. The *Neijing Suwen* tells us that "the Eastern quarter produces wind and wind produces Wood."[5] The Chinese character for *dong* 东 east contains the character *mu* for Wood and the character *ri* for sun. The graphic depicts the sun rising through the branches of a tree in the early morning. For the ancient Chinese, the east is the quarter of the yang qi, the quarter of the rising sun, the arousing of green life in Spring and the morning time of the annual *sheng* cycle. The association between Wood and east offers a clue to the nature of Wood's spirit and points to a link between Wood, wind, trees, clouds, sky, light and the *hun* soul's capacity for creative vision, effective planning and growth in accordance with Tao.

The *hun* is the spirit of vision and imagination. It is the aspect of our psyche that presides over our dreams and our capacity to plan, hope and move forward into new possibilities. The *hun* soul endows us with the capacity for decisiveness and direction for our life, the ability to go to our own edge and stay on track, to plan and organize our time in order to manifest our vision. It allows us to sleep well and open to dreams that guide us in the outer world and help us know our inner world more deeply.

The *hun* is comprised of a trio of souls: Dark Essence, Brilliance of the Fetus and Clear Spiritual Force. All three are said to reside in the eyes by day and to descend to rest in the Liver by night. Their day/night, up/down rhythm connects the dark essences of the Kidneys, the *zhi* and lower body with the clear spiritual force of the Heart, the *shen* and the mind. Through this connection between Water and Fire, the light of the spiritual embryo is ignited within us.

Together, the three *hun* preside over the pineal and pituitary glands that regulate growth and sleep, and all aspects of our being that have to do with the awareness, reception and metabolism of light and images. The *hun* direct our imaginative functions and our capacity to "see" into our own future, to envision new possibilities and to plan scenarios through which these possibilities can be realized.

In essence, the *hun* support us as we find our path through the infinite possibilities and decisions of life. They allow us to go our own way while staying in right relationship to the world around us and to shout out the great "I am" of becoming who we are truly meant to be.

Wood's spirit question: To what degree am I growing and developing toward my ultimate purpose or destiny?

Spirit Animal: The Green Dragon

It is said that, "long ago, the dragon began as a winged or flying serpent, expressing the primal harmony between the subterranean and aerial dimensions."[6] The Green Dragon is the spirit of the Wood Element. His given name is Dragon Smoke. His secret name is Hidden Clarity because he allows us to see where we are going. His color is *qing* 青 blue-green or azure, the color of nature, Spring and growing plants. Within the Chinese character used to indicate the special color *qing*, we find *sheng* 生 life and *dan* 丹 alchemy. The Green Dragon's color tells us something about its special alchemical, renewing and life-giving capacities along with the alchemical, vitalizing nature of the green world itself.

The Green Dragon is not the fearsome, devouring monster of Greek mythology and European medieval legends. Rather, the Green Dragon is a harbinger and protector of new life. He is an emblem of guardianship and vigilance and brings courage and strength in the face of challenge.

The Green Dragon is associated with arousing yang energy, the quickening that comes at the end of winter, the virile fertility of the plant world and the possibility of resurrection and renewal. With the arrival of spring, the Green Dragon wakes from his sleep, crawls out from his mountain cavern lair, rises from the riverbeds and marshes to spread his greenness over the Earth. We hear his voice in the rumbling of spring thunderstorms that come as he races up into the sky.

The Green Dragon is directly connected to the first hexagram of the *I Ching*, The Creative - *Ch'ien*, whose six unbroken yang lines stand for the "primal power, which is light-giving, active, strong and of the spirit."[7]

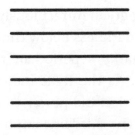

HEXAGRAM 1 - THE CREATIVE - *CH'IEN*

In addition to his yang virility, the Green Dragon is endowed with a special power to move between worlds, to link Above and Below by descending deep into the Watery depths of the Earth and then rising to the Fiery heights of Heaven. The commentary on the changing lines of the hexagram describes the full circle of the Green Dragon's yearly journey as he rises up from the underworld with the Wood Element in Spring and drops back down at the closing of Late Summer.[8] If we look with the eyes of the imagination, we can see him climb the ladder of the hexagram from Below to Above and then back again.

The first and lowest line of the hexagram represents Winter, the time when the Green Dragon withdraws beneath the ground to hibernate in the darkness. The Green Dragon is invisible. Green life disappears from the world as trees lose their leaves, vegetation dies and the life force sinks down into the roots and seeds beneath the ground.

The second line represents the arousing of the Green Dragon as he awakens from hibernation, breaks through the darkness of the underworld and appears in the fields as the first sprouting of seeds of spring. As the light and warmth of the yang increase, the Green Dragon opens his wild eyes and begins to move. Like a clap of thunder, he rises from beneath the dark soil. As his great flanks emerge from the underworld, vegetation spreads across the fields and forests. A skin of shimmering green miraculously sprouts from seeds buried in the unseen darkness below the ground.

The third line marks a period of transition from yin to yang, low to high. As the light increases and the Green Dragon continues to rise, his power to ignite, activate and illuminate increases. The third line impresses the importance of balancing the Green Dragon's outer yang activity with the inner yin resources he has gathered and cultivated through his rest in the darkness as he moves between hiddenness and visibility and as the energies of the *sheng* cycle move from the incubation and gestation of Water to the visioning and birthing of Wood.

The fourth line represents the Green Dragon's first wavering flight above the dark depths. As Spring progresses, the Green Dragon tentatively flexes his wings. The green color rises up from the grass to the hedgerows and then the tops of the trees. The world is still in transition between the Winter and Summer, Water and Fire. It's up to the Green Dragon to decide which way to fly, to take the right course, to forward the great cycle of the year and maintain the balance of the Tao.

Then it happens! It's Summer and the Green Dragon ascends. The fifth line represents the "flying Dragon in the heavens."[9] Leaving behind the ripening green-gold meadows, he spreads open his vast wings and lifts his heavy body into the brilliant summer sky. Up and over the moon, he flies his water-born serpent's body into the Heavenly lights. Now we see him as a ball of fire, a yellow orb of sunlight in the vast distance, shining out across the lands, and the *I Ching* tells us, "Thus the sage arises, and all creatures follow him with their eyes."[10]

At last, in Late Summer, gravity and entropy prevail and the Green Dragon's great body begins to weigh him down. The sixth line represents the turning point when yin emerges again from yang, when all the solid, unbroken yang lines of the first hexagram, the Creative - *Ch'ien*, break and transform to the second hexagram, the Receptive - *K'un*.

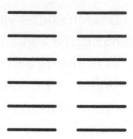

HEXAGRAM 2 - THE RECEPTIVE - *K'UN*

Now, "the strength of the Creative and the mildness of the Receptive unite."[11] At the apex of his ascent, trailing plumes of smoke, the power of his bright yang head tucked beneath his dark yin wing, humbled and worn but undaunted, the Green Dragon falls. Hiding his great strength, mild in his manner and accepting the inevitable pull of the yin, he descends back to his home in the deep waters, bringing the blessings of rain and messages from the stars.

The Green Dragon symbolizes the Wood Element's yang energy that rises in Spring and rushes upward toward the light. We know that it takes a lot of energy to lift such a huge animal into the sky—the qi of the entire *sheng* cycle goes into this lifting—so the Green Dragon has the most negentropy of all the spirit animals. In the inner world, he represents the power of the creative imagination to free us from the limiting bonds of Earth, to counterbalance gravity and the weight of matter, to lift us up into the stars where we can hear the messages of spirit, and then descend again to manifest our Tao and do our work of making the invisible visible, the possible real.

The Green Dragon is the protector of the eastern direction. We call on the Green Dragon when it's time to rise, time to move with the wild impetuous growth impulses of the Wood element. The Green Dragon stands by our side and gives us the courage we need to move forward on the explorations and adventures of life. We call on the Green Dragon to protect us on our visionary journeys. We depend on him to accompany us as we enter the realm of dreams. He is the guardian of the *hun*, of the cinnabar caves, of the lifeblood that rushes through our bodies and of all the parts of our being that perceive the light. We rely on him to give us the power to fly, to temporarily reverse the limiting bonds of time, space and matter so that we can catch a glimpse of the infinite possibilities that lie beyond.

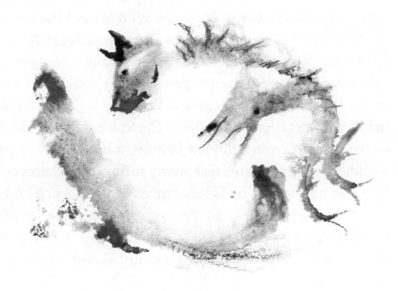

GREEN DRAGON

Archetype: The Green Man

Long ago, in a time that we know through our dreams and our twilight longing for the green world, human beings lived in the woods. They feasted on acorns and freely growing fruit and slept in silver nests of leaves facing upwards toward the moon. The Norse words *bua* and *bowen*, from which our word "bough" is derived, originally meant "to dwell," and these roots pull us back into that time when we were dwellers in the boughs of trees, when we were gently rocked by the wind and washed by rain. As tree-dwellers we were long muscled, tenacious and sinewy yet supple and lithe. We reached our arms upward with graceful determination toward the open sky and sank our feet down deep into the cool, dark soil. The memory of trees that is reflected in the shape of our bodies and the vision of our souls is the legacy of the Wood Element. This legacy lives in us as an archetype, and this archetype is personified by the Green Man, the Wild Man of the Woods.

The Green Man is related to the vegetative deities that spring up in different cultures throughout the ages. This archetype represents the irrepressible, sly and joyous nature of the life force. He expresses the unity that exists between man and vegetation and reflects the universality of the laws of nature that govern human beings, animals and the green world. The Green Man takes many forms, but wherever and however he appears, he is recognized as the horned god, the joyous drunken dancer of Spring, the yang energy of the astrological sign Aries; the personification of yang male fertility, boundless hope, new possibilities, wild wisdom and lusty desire.

The Green Man often appears as a human head, immersed in foliage. We come across him on the plinths and pillars of old stone churches in the British Isles and northern Europe, on the side of a shed in an overgrown garden or staring out at us from the gnarled bark of a tree, especially when the light is dim. Sometimes vegetation is growing out of his mouth, eyes and ears, often enfolding his face so that we are uncertain whether he is made of flesh or vine, whether red blood or green chlorophyll flows through his veins. Gazing out from the wild snake-like proliferation of vinery, the eyes of the Green Man disturb, delight and seduce us. We're confused and unable to discern what is human and what is vegetative, and we're reminded of our original oneness with the soil, our connection and interdependence with nature and the green nation.

When asked if he believed that a tree was a kind of entity, botanist, redwood tree climber and Green Man Steve Sillett replied that a tree is "a being. It's a 'person,' from a plant's point of view. A tree is not conscious, the way we are, but it has a perfect memory...it begins life the same way we do, with a sperm and an egg...is responsive and alive. Trees react more slowly than we do, but see how intricate they become."[12]

Tom Bombadil, the mysterious Green Man of J. R. R. Tolkien's *The Fellowship of the Ring*, also speaks of the forest as a being apart from us. He reminds us that "the Old Forest is the ancient survivor of vast forgotten woods"[13] that at one time covered all the continents of the Earth. In the Old Forest, Tom Bombadil tells of the fathers of the fathers of trees, the Great Willow. The Green Willow's "heart was rotten but his strength was green; and he was cunning, and a master of winds, and his song and thought ran through the woods on both sides of the river. His grey thirsty spirit drew power out of the earth and spread like fine root threads in the ground, and invisible twig-fingers in the air, till it had under its dominion nearly all the trees of the Forest from the Hedge to the Downs."[14] These are the old forests where our dream bodies go to dwell at night and drift in the vine-covered arms of the Green Man.

Alchemy: Transforming Force into Flow

Crucial to a healthy relationship with Wood is harmony and balance. In order to carry out its function as the directing agent of new possibilities, the Wood must not only be determined and directed, it must also have fluidity and flexibility to adapt to the needs of others as well as the conditions of the environment. Without the alchemical tension of opposites between hard and soft, turgid and flexible, directed and flowing, the Wood is not able to bring the inherent possibility of the Tao into manifest form. So in the Spring season or any time the Wood is in ascendancy in our life, it is important to temper activity with rest, to restore our bodies and minds with adequate sleep and to replenish our blood with nutrient-rich greens. The Wood invites us to take the time to plan and vision before we act and to be willing to flow around obstacles rather than exhausting our resources in a direct assault against them. Whenever possible, the wisdom of Wood counsels flow rather than force, poetry rather than rant and benevolent vision rather than angry attack.

Wood Spirit Points

Gall Bladder 13 - Root of the Spirit - *Ben Shen*

本 神

It comes suddenly
this memory of Spring, like tears
that thaw a frozen heart.

First there is nothing. Then, an excitation, not yet visible to the eye yet felt by the body. And then, here and there where the snow has melted, the first courageous sprouts of green emerge. A bedraggled robin returns. Birch buds swell. The light brightens. The thunder of newly stirring growth can be faintly heard from deep below the earth. The Green Dragon opens one sleepy eye and begins to rise.

Gall Bladder 13 - Root of the Spirit - *Ben Shen* 本 神 is a point that resonates with this time in early Spring when the cosmic wheel turns from yin to yang and the world is suspended in a momentary breathless balance. On the horary cycle of the Chinese clock, Gall Bladder time (11pm–1am) occurs directly across from the time of the Heart (11am–1pm). The Heart marks the turning point of the day, at noon, when the maximum forces of yang turn to yin. The Gall Bladder marks the turning point of the night, at midnight, when the maximum forces of yin turn to yang. Taken together, these two officials function as pivot points around which the twin lights of Heaven, the sun and the moon, revolve, just as yin and yang revolve around the central axis of the *tai ji* symbol ☯. Root of the Spirit - *Ben Shen* is the command point for this fulcrum, a point we can turn to when the inner axis has become wobbly due to shock, trauma, loss or radical changes in a person's life.

The character for Gall Bladder 胆 includes the radical *dan* 旦 which is a picture of the sun rising up over the horizon. The character reiterates the Gall Bladder's function as an agent of illumination, the official who turns the darkness back to light. However, the character for Gall Bladder 胆 is also used to mean courage, the quality of daring audacity that we recognize in the yang brightness of the sun at dawn.

As an affirmation of its unique capacity for bravery, the Gall Bladder is the only one of the *fu* or yang hollow organs to have its own unique spirit animal, a curious mythical creature, part turtle, part snake, who is known as the True Warrior. On the outside, the True Warrior is strongly defended by a hard shell. On the inside, he is soft, quick, sinuous and shrewd. The creature's name is Majestic Clarity and his image appears on the protective shields of shamans and other spiritual warriors. His special function is to protect the Heart and root the light of the *shen*.

Another significant aspect of the Gall Bladder is that it stores bile, a clear golden yellow elixir that empowers digestive processes and is considered by Taoist alchemists to be the root of terrestrial or post-natal life. On the physical level, it promotes the digestion of food. On the level of spirit, it helps us "digest" experiences so that we can move on, particularly when shock or trauma has resulted in chronic states of fear or timidity. This spirit-level digestive capacity is strengthened in Root of the Spirit - *Ben Shen* by its connection to the *Yang Wei* channel, which functions to help us digest impressions in order to bring our outer experiences into the body. At the same time, it also encourages us to let go of unnecessary attachments and "move on when one is stuck in cycles of time."[15]

Root of the Spirit - *Ben Shen* integrates the Gall Bladder's digestive function with its capacity for wise judgment and appropriate timing so that we can assess the current conditions and decide on the next step. It activates our fierce protectiveness when necessary and our courageous audacity when the moment is right. It is a point that is especially useful when shock or trauma has dislodged the *shen* from its rooting in the Heart, resulting in debilitating hesitancy and timidity, disorientation and disconnection from Tao.

Like the branches of a tree that reach up to the sun, the Gall Bladder channel opens to Heaven through *Ben Shen*. The point gathers up the light of scattered spirit as it metabolizes and transforms experience and memory into useable nutrients for the soul. As experience is transformed into wisdom, the darkness of night is illuminated by consciousness and the *shen* returns to its proper rooting in the Heart.

The point is recognized for its value in the treatment of headaches, visual dizziness and neck tightness, but these physical-level symptoms are indicative of only the most superficial aspects of the point's true nature. The point has strong psychological and spirit-level effects and can be a key ally when addressing psycho-spiritual issues in the treatment room. An important aspect of the Gall Bladder's effect on the psyche has to do with its capacity to instill courage—the capacity to move us forward in the face of challenges. Thus, psychological indicators for this point include fear, extreme upset, out-of-control behavior and hysteria. It's especially useful for children who are timid or frightened. In addition, it can be used for unreasonable feelings of jealousy, paranoia, worry and states of disassociation—all situations where the fulcrum or central axis of life has become unhinged.

As the pivotal organ on the nocturnal side of the Chinese clock, Root of the Spirit - *Ben Shen* functions as a connecting link between yin and yang. Key to the spirit purpose of this point is the maintenance of the balance of the emotional life—the capacity to know, judge and decide when to move forward and when to rest. As the connecting link between night and day, yin and yang, it supports the rooting of the yang energies of the *hun* in the yin essences of the body. When the *hun* is well rooted in the Liver and the blood, the visions, plans and blueprints of the Liver can be brought down into concrete form by the decisions of the Gall Bladder and the steps that it implements. Root of the Spirit - *Ben Shen* helps us to decide—to know—the right turn to take at each fork in the road as it roots the light of the *shen* in the daily movements of our life.

Suggested Flower Essence: Star of Bethlehem

I have found that the application of flower essences to acupuncture points is especially effective for points located on the head, neck and ears. I believe that this is due to the strong affinity between the yang, highly refined vibration of the essences and the mind and spirit. Due to this vibrational affinity, the right essence can have an immediate effect on the mental and emotional body and the Heart, calming the spirit and making way for further reorganizing and reorienting to authentic nature.

Star of Bethlehem is one of the essences I often turn to when a person's *shen* has become uprooted by shock or trauma, whether from a recent event or an inadequately resolved incident from the past. The medicine of this Heavenly blue six-petaled flower helps to restore coherence and rhythm to the nervous system and allow a person to gradually recover awareness of emotions that have been buried beneath a protective wall of numbness and rigidity. In addition, it clears foggy, trauma-muddled memories so that we can once again connect with the renewing energies of source and origin.

When applied to Root of the Spirit - *Ben Shen*, I have found that star of Bethlehem augments the point's capacity to root the *shen*. It helps to reunify mind and heart when they have disassociated in an attempt to survive unbearable experiences. Most importantly, it activates the Gall Bladder's capacity to digest experiences, to appropriately protect and defend the vulnerability of the Heart and to act with valor and courage when these qualities are called for. When timidity, anxiety and distrust have become habitual protective strategies, a drop of star of Bethlehem on *Ben Shen* can help to restore my sense of safety and connection to inner divinity that allows me to shine the light of my true self out into the world. As the clouds of numbness and disassociation clear, I once again perceive the light of my own North Star and find my way back to the path of Tao.

Gall Bladder 16 - Window of the Eye - *Mu Chuang* 目窗

Look now, how the red
head of the woodpecker lights up
this rainy morning.

Like the woodpecker pecking trees in search of nesting holes in spring, the qi movement induced by a needle in Gall Bladder 16 - Window of the Eye - *Mu Chuang* 目窗 is not subtle or slow. The energy here is strong and determined. Needling this point is a quick, clear call for rebirth and change. I turn to this point when a person is ready to open to something new. When an old way of being is no longer relevant or a period of long gestation is complete, this point supports clear vision and allows us to "see" where and how our life wants to grow. After banging our heads against the same closed door, this point opens a window and reminds us that the world is not a linear, black-and-white design but rather a multifaceted array of tones, colors and choices.

Although the currently accepted applications of this point are limited to a few physical symptoms located in the head, including dizziness, superficial visual obstruction, eye swelling, nasal congestion and early stages of colds,[16] I have found it to be an invaluable ally when clarity of vision, whether on the physical or spirit level, has become impaired. Just as we instinctively fling open the window to better see the beauty of an early spring morning, we open the Eye Window to better see the possibilities of our lives.

The name of the point Window of the Eye - *Mu Chuang* 目窗 combines a stylized picture of an eye *mu* 目—a pupil and eyelids turned sideways—with *chuang* 窗, which combines the radical *xue* 穴, a hole, cave or acupuncture point, with the phonetic *chuang* 囪, a picture of a skylight or window. The point's name affirms our understanding of its ability to open us to the light, particularly light that comes down from above. In spirit-level terms, I consider it to be a passageway for the *hun*, the spirit of the Wood Element, the eyes and the messengers of the *shen*.

As I open to the Heavenly illumination that shines through my open Eye Window, my dreams become clearer and more meaningful. My imagination is enlivened, and my capacity to see a hopeful future is renewed. In the words of acupuncturist and scholar Debra Kaatz, "At *Mu Chuang* our vision opens and life sparkles. We are suddenly able to see the fullness of life in every detail that surrounds us."[17]

Suggested Flower Essence: Clary Sage

Clary sage essential oil has a wide variety of medicinal properties. From a traditional Chinese medicine perspective, it clears deficiency heat, subdues Liver wind and circulates stagnant qi. In addition, it has a unique capacity to harmonize and balance. Depending on need, it acts as either a stimulant or a relaxant. The oil can be used as a tonic in cases of mental fatigue but also as a sedative when the mind is overstimulated.

On a spirit level, the inner wisdom of this oil also has a balancing nature that lies in its capacity to open a person to their inner and outer vision. Gabriel Mojay reminds us that the word *clary* "is derived from the Latin word *clarus* meaning clear—reflecting the role of this oil in treating eye complaints."[18] For our purposes, we are particularly interested in its ability to clear away the mists that cloud our inner vision.

I apply a drop of clary sage to Window of the Eye - *Mu Chuang* when I want to open the window of the soul. By calming the mind and lifting the spirit, this treatment invites a realistic hopefulness along with clarity about one's purpose and direction. Where there is muddled thinking and confusion about the next step or an upcoming decision, I find that this oil can help a person to see clearly what they could not see before. When the Eye Window is open and enlivened by the healing properties of this sacred oil, we see with our "owl's eyes," the eyes of inner wisdom, and the night is illuminated by the shining of the spirit.

A caveat: clary sage is an estrogenic oil. It should not be used during pregnancy or in cases where there are hormone sensitivity issues.

Gall Bladder 24 - Sun and Moon - *Ri Yue*

日月

Spring equinox. Twilight.
The sun dips down behind my back
as I greet the rising moon.

Gall Bladder 24 - Sun and Moon - *Ri Yue* 日月 expresses the energy of the fleeting moment when the cosmic principals of yin and yang pause in perfect balance at the equinox. As the season turns from winter to spring, day and night come into equilibrium. This is a time to open to the darkness and the light, our lunar and our solar vision, our inner and our outer knowing. Just as the sun and the moon both shine in the twilight sky at the spring full moon, so our two ways of knowing can be present to us simultaneously without one dimming or obliterating the other.

When we combine the character *ri* 日 sun with *yue* 月 moon, we create *ming* 明. *Ming* is commonly translated to mean bright and also sight, clear and intelligent understanding. But for the ancient Taoists, the word had deeper philosophical and spiritual implications and was used to mean spiritual illumination and enlightenment. For traditional physicians, the light of the sun and the moon joining together in this point "describe the quality of judgment emanating from a healthy Gall Bladder."[19]

At the physical level, Sun and Moon - *Ri Yue* is traditionally recognized for its ability to treat a wide variety of eye disorders, including redness, swelling and superficial obstruction and visual dizziness.[20] But on a spirit level, I cherish the point for its inner gift, its capacity to balance the yin and yang aspects of the soul and, in particular, the connection it engenders between our inner visions and dreams and the plans we make and actions we take in the outer world.

The quality of courage, the ability to stand our ground and the willingness to face and speak our own truth are all characteristics of a healthy Gall Bladder. Sun and Moon - *Ri Yue* is a spirit point that will support these capacities as it brings us closer to our own integrity and wholeness and allows us to embrace both our extroversion and introversion, action and receptivity, speech and silence.

Suggested Treatment Strategy: Connecting Physical and Spirit-Level Aspects of the Gall Bladder Official

A young woman recovering from serious orthopedic surgery on a congenital deformation of her left hip socket comes into my office before leaving to visit a former lover and to consider renewing their relationship. The scar line runs directly through the Gall Bladder line at Gall Bladder 30 - Jumping Circle - *Huan Tiao*.

"I feel so different after the surgery. My brain feels fuzzy, as if I can't think straight. I can't keep multiple things in focus the way I did before the surgery." She pauses, then adds, "I am afraid that I won't know how to deal with intimacy anymore. I don't know how I am going to respond or what I am going to need."

She is afraid of stepping out into the world again. She is, as she says, shaky on her new feet.

Gradually, we identify that her Gall Bladder is having trouble working out all the details of her trip and she is having anxiety about the uncertainty. The radical reorganizing of structures resulting from the surgery, specifically along the course of the Gall Bladder meridian, has also resulted in a psycho-spiritual reorganization, a shift in the Gall Bladder Official's capacity to make the decisions necessary to implement not only the details of her road trip but also her life plan. The congenital abnormality that resulted in compensations on a physical level also affected her psychologically. These psychological compensations included an over-reliance on mental functioning, compulsive management of details and the useful but constricting need to have her future under control. But now, all this is changing.

As my patient comes to understand that her surgery has affected not only her body but also her psyche, she opens to the possibility that the shift may have a very positive effect on her emotional and her physical wellbeing. She recognizes that despite the discomfort involved in any process of radical change, there can also be great benefits. Together, we agree that the new possibility for her is the capacity to listen to the needs of her own body and to make decisions based on her deeper needs rather than on external demands and collective values. A new attitude of caring for her interior life is replacing her old way of compulsively pushing beyond her own limits.

After doing other work on more physical aspects of her recovery, I decide to needle Sun and Moon - *Ri Yue* as a spirit point, a way to support her in opening to a more balanced way of looking at her life. Before I needle the point, we talk about how she may need to slow down, to take time to go in and listen in a new way to her body, honoring the more yin lunar wisdom within as well as her outer yang solar intellect. We talk about how the receptivity of inner yin vision complements, softens and deepens the penetrating active nature of outer yang clarity and sight. She begins to consider the real possibility that she can trust the wisdom of her body to guide her actions in the outer world.

I needle the point, and she closes her eyes and rests for a while. After I remove the needle and check her pulses, she sits up.

"I feel different," she says. "I really get it. A lot has changed for me. Why would I respond in the way I did before when I am not that same person? I'm feeling energy move through my body and I actually feel excited. It's time for me to get back out there and see who I am now."

Her eyes are bright and shining with presence, clarity and depth. There it is, I think, the light of the sun and the moon, *ming*—a new and different light to guide her on the journey.

Gall Bladder 37 - Bright and Clear - *Guang Ming*
光明

As if morning clouds
had been erased, a streak of gold
lights up this painted sky.

The illuminating nature of this Gall Bladder point is expressed by the point name. Just as we find in the name of the previous point (Gall Bladder 24 - Sun and Moon - *Ri Yue*), Gall Bladder 37 - Bright and Clear - *Guang Ming* 光明 includes the radicals of the sun and moon as well as the keyword *ming* 明 used by Taoists to refer to spiritual enlightenment and clarity of mind. Here, however, we find the addition of the character *guang* 光—a picture of *ren* 人 a person carrying a torch of *huo* 火 fire. *Guang* is translated as light, brightness and luster. It can also be used to mean a kind of graciousness of manner, honor or glory.

The important physical-level applications of this point are widely recognized and include standard Gall Bladder symptoms such as eye issues, one-sided headaches, jaw tightness and breast tenderness (through its *luo* connection to the Liver and sinew channel links with the breasts). I would add my own experience of its value in the treatment of one-sided eye twitching. Additionally, the point is known for its ability to treat local symptoms such as knee pain and various other disorders in the lower legs.

However, my reverence for the power of this point is not for its many physical uses but rather for its ability to radically alter and harmonize the emotions. Like all the other *luo*-connecting points, this point has a special affinity with the emotional body. In my experience, Bright and Clear - *Guang*

Ming can act as a powerful magic wand of grace. When this point is called for, it may be the only one I need in order to effect the necessary shift at the spirit level.

In the standard list of indications, there is generally mention of the use of Bright and Clear - *Guang Ming* for the treatment of unruly emotions such as irascibility and "sudden mania."[21] Here is where I find its genius! This point does much more than clarify the vision and open the eyes. It can also be used to treat emotional lability, chronic frustration, anger and inappropriate aggression. It calms stress and spasming and unbinds stagnation on physical, emotional and spiritual levels. When we access the spirit-level wisdom of this point, it offers an illumination that can penetrate the haze of whatever upsets we are experiencing. As the wildfires of hyperactivity, anxiety, anger and rage are subdued, we return to *ming*, to our own radiance of spirit.

Then we once again can walk with grace, with the torch of our inner light held steady in our hands.

Suggested Treatment Strategy: Harnessing the Power of the Point

Bright and Clear - *Guang Ming* is a powerful point that requires strong and intentional needling in order to do its magic. In my experience, this is not a point that responds to a flower essence or gentle touch. Its nature is more of lightning and dragons than mists and whispers. This means I am going to be diligent in point location and do the point again if I do not activate the qi. I bring the full force of my Gall Bladder True Warrior energy to my intention, needle in the direction of the flow of the meridian and look for streaming sensations that move down into the foot. Surprisingly, even my most sensitive, needle-shy patients respond favorably to this kind of needling on this point, as the welcome, harmonizing shifts and illuminations it brings are immediately palpable.

Gall Bladder 41 - Foot Above Tears - *Zu Lin Qi*
足臨泣

I stand at the edge
of Water and Wood. Waiting
for approaching Spring.

At winter's end, I stand at the edge of the garden, looking out at the exposed beds, the brown fallen leaves and the bare tree branches, wondering how this muddy patch of ground could ever come back to life, to the riot of color and green vitality I remember from previous years. But as I am about to turn back inside, I look down. Just there, where a small pool of melting snow has gathered at the base of the old maple, I see the green shoots. And then the white teardrops of the flowers...a clump of tiny snowdrops at my feet...the very first signs of spring.

Gall Bladder 41 - Foot Above Tears - *Zu Lin Qi* 足臨泣 embodies the energy of sprouting snowdrops in early spring. When I first learned about this point, I liked the name for both its poetry and its strangeness. I quickly came to appreciate the power of the point, including it in my earliest point palette. I welcomed its direct Wood-within-Wood nature, its ability to regulate the breath, calm the emotions and shift diaphragmatic holding patterns by releasing the constricting belt of the *Dai Mo*. I found that opening the flow of qi between Foot Above Tears - *Zu Lin Qi* and Liver 1 - Great Esteem - *Da Dun* generally had a positive effect on a constrained Wood Element and could often help resolve issues related to dampness and obstruction in the legs.

But still I wondered about the point name. What could it be telling me about the spirit-level nature of this point?

Many years later, I found a clue. At the heart of the three-part point name is the character *lin* 臨, a picture of a wide-eyed person looking out over some small objects at her feet. The original ancient character looked like this:

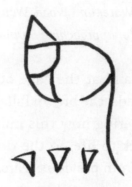

ANCIENT GRAPHIC: *LIN*

There's me. Looking down at three snowdrops sprouting at my feet. But there's more. *Lin* is also the title of Hexagram 19 of the *I Ching*. In the text, Richard Wilhelm translates the word *lin* as "approach." However, he writes in the commentary:

> The Chinese word *lin* has a range of meanings that is not exhausted by any single word of another language. The ancient explanation...is "becoming great." What becomes great are the two strong lines growing into the hexagram from below; the light-giving power expands with them...this hexagram is linked with the twelfth month, when, after the winter solstice, the light power begins to ascend again.[22]

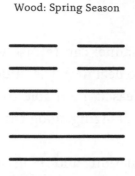

HEXAGRAM 19 - APPROACH - *LIN*

Meditating further on the hexagram, I discover that it focuses not only on the joyous, hopeful progress of approaching spring but also on the importance of perseverance and determination, both qualities of a healthy Gall Bladder. If we are to make the most of the moment and the tendency toward movement and change that are implied by the rising yang lines, we must seize the day and be prepared for fearless action. Timing is of the utmost importance and, as Wilhelm's commentary reminds us, "spring does not last forever."[23] If we act in the right way, with the right attitude, at the right time, evil can be averted before it has "even begun to stir."[24]

Here again, we find the crucial significance of the Gall Bladder's capacity for right timing and courageous action when the moment calls for it. The radical *qi* 泣 tears is actually a picture of *li* 立, a person standing on the ground, next to *shui* 氵, an oncoming wave of water. The point invites us to stand tall and rise above possible threats of the oncoming wave of dangers and uncertainties and, like a sprouting seed in spring, dare to move audaciously toward the light.

The inner meaning is affirmed by the fact that Foot Above Tears - *Zu Lin Qi* is the master opening point of *Dai Mo*, the belt meridian that encircles the waistline. Acupuncturist and Doctor of Oriental Medicine David Twicken reminds us that "the Dai is about not being able to deal with things in the now. The Dai channel can release what we have stored, allowing the space to deal with the underlying conditions."[25] When the belt is released, I am able to exhale, let go of the baggage I have been dragging along through the long winter and be on the move.

Dampness, stagnation and constraint are the main accumulations that plague the *Dai Mo* channel. When, due to excessive caution and fear, I resist the natural tendency of the Wood Element to metabolize experiences and move forward into life, dampness accumulates. But when I surrender to the currents of life in spring, dampness transforms and the flowing Water can nourish new growth. Tears are the natural outpouring of the soul when we let go of the past and step forward to approach our future.

Liver 3 - Supreme Rushing - *Tai Chong*
太衝

Ice melts and water
gushes up. Between black stones
wild cress sprouts green.

Suddenly, the senses open and light, sound and color return to the world. All that has been bound and constricted begins again to move. Snow melts into rivulets and mud puddles. Goldfinches return to the cedar tree, turkeys roam in search of early bugs and a mating pair of red-tailed squirrels run in circles around the trunk of the apple tree. This is the energy of early spring, a time of exuberant expansion, aggressive desire and an almost mad frenzy of activity as the yang qi moves back into ascendancy. The sky opens as the sun returns, ready to wake the world, to shift the pitch of light, to give the go-ahead, the green light, the big "yes" that signals the buds to swell, seeds to sprout and eggs to hatch.

Liver 3 - Supreme Rushing - *Tai Chong* 太衝 is the archetype, the primary code point, of early spring. It moves us from the slow, gestational containing energies of Water into the liberated enthusiasm of the Wood Element. Nestled deep in the crook, at the meeting point of the metatarsals of the first and second toes, this point opens the gateway for the energy of Wood. In much the same way that warming temperatures and returning sunlight bring movement, vitality and the vibrant assertion of life back to the world after the quiescent dormancy of winter, Supreme Rushing - *Tai Chong* brings easeful flow, hope and healthy aggression back to the body, soul and spirit. When there is frustration, constraint, rigidity, repressed anger or a sense of impediment to taking a necessary leap into the next phase of a journey, this point is a powerful ally.

As the Earth Point on the Liver meridian, Supreme Rushing - *Tai Chong* offers the nourishment and rooting that the Wood Element needs in order to sprout upward and grow with stability, vigor and power. As source, the point is also adaptogenic. In other words, it knows what is needed. It can be used to sedate, cool and calm overly activated Liver yang or tonify, warm and motivate Liver yin. It can nourish the Liver blood when deficient and de-constrain it when stagnant.

Supreme Rushing - *Tai Chong* is another of Ma Danyang's Twelve Heavenly Star Points.[26] In his commentary on this point, the ancient physician tells us that "lowering the needle brings magical results."[27] Danyang notes that Supreme Rushing - *Tai Chong* cures fits and convulsions, relieves swelling of throat and breasts, is helpful for all types of hernias and alleviates one-sided drooping and heaviness and aching in the waist due to qi stagnation.

In addition, Danyang writes of the point's ability to "disperse cloudy mists in front of the eyes and restore movement when the two feet are unable to walk."[28] On a physical level, this application reinforces the point's importance for the treatment of "blurriness and cloudy vision" and "flaccidity of legs and inability to walk."[29] I believe that "cloudy mists in front of the eyes" could also be interpreted to mean a lack of inner vision and clarity of plans and purpose on a spirit level. Without vision and plans, our life path is uncertain and it is impossible to manifest the Divine mandate of our life. We stumble or feel completely unable to move forward on the journey of our Tao. This deeper, psycho-spiritual meaning is affirmed when I look more closely at the point name.

The character *chong* 衝 is composed of two radicals. The first—*xing* 行—is a picture of two footprints and means to walk. The second phonetic—*chong* 重—is a picture of a pile of flat weights on a weighing machine and refers to something that has weight, heft and importance. *Chong* can also imply value and a kind of power or potency of effect. The special potency of the forward movement activated by the point is emphasized by the qualifying word *tai* 太 meaning supreme or great. At the deepest level, the name tells me that Supreme Rushing - *Tai Chong* activates a clarity of vision and purpose that allows for empowered movement forward into my life. Like a healthy green sprout in early spring, I follow my path through the darkness toward the light and grow, without hesitation or doubt, into the fullest possible expression of my authentic nature.

Suggested Treatment Strategy: Connecting Supreme Rushing -
Tai Chong *and Kidney 1 - Bubbling Spring -* Yong Guan

Supreme Rushing - *Tai Chong* was the first point I ever had needled and the experience was so powerful that it changed the course of my life. As the needle penetrated my skin and sank into the hollow between the bones of my foot, I felt a powerful surge of energy rush through me and then deep relaxation. The veil that had been covering my senses lifted. The world cracked open and light rained like water through my body. Although it took me another year of treatment to recognize that my destiny was to become an acupuncturist, the opening of the vision and the initial impulse of the plan originated with the rush of *de qi* that streamed through my body in response to the skillful needling of this point.

Due to its adaptogenic nature and its multiplicity of effects, it is crucial that my intention is crystal clear when I needle this point. Before inserting the needle, I need to know where and how I want the Liver qi to flow. Gentle needling against the direction of meridian and retention of the needle will result in the sedation of the Liver—the release of irritability, frustration and stress and calming of an over-activated *hun*. Stronger, more assertive needling in the direction of flow along with rice grain moxa will activate the Liver and nourish and move the blood. It is also at times appropriate to choose a neutral insertion, placing the needle in an upright position, retaining it without any additional stimulation and allowing it to find its own relationship to the qi when there are signs of excess with underlying deficiency.

Another technique that is particularly useful for treating cloudiness of vision is needling Supreme Rushing - *Tai Chong* in tandem with Bubbling Spring - *Yong Guan*. This combination is especially valuable when a person cannot "see" a hopeful future, has no sense of purpose and is unable to walk forward toward their destiny. When we connect Bubbling Spring - *Yong Guan* to Supreme Rushing - *Tai Chong*, we call upon the exuberant energies of melting ice and snow in late winter to nourish the new green growth of early spring. The light and animating power of the yang is increased and clarity of sight is restored. The two feet can once again walk without stumbling and, seemingly "by magic," one's path is revealed.

Liver 5 - Insect Ditch - *Li Gou*
蠡溝

Transformers of soil.
Blossom blessers. Pond wakers. Back biters.
Bugs! Rejoice! It's Spring!

And then, one day, the tipping point overturns and spring gets hot! Overnight, the golden dandelions become puffballs of flying seeds. The tender lettuces wilt in the midday sun. The irises swell on their stalks and tumble headfirst on top of the peonies. Wood's power of thrusting, birthing, growing and unfolding has resulted in an abundance of life that can barely keep up with itself. And following right on schedule after the rain, sunlight and burgeoning vegetation comes the creeping, crawling, whirling, whizzing buzz of bugs!

Liver 5 - Insect Ditch - *Li Gou* 蠡溝 is a point that addresses issues of excess in the Liver channel. I turn to this point when the exuberant creativity of the Wood Element has gotten out of hand, resulting in problems such as itching, swelling, distension, inflexibility, discharge and stagnation, as well as retention of urine, plum stone qi and incessant erections! In other words, this is the point to use when the Wood Element has too much to process and metabolize and the life force needs support to get things moving smoothly again.

Insect Ditch - *Li Gou* acts like a fresh spring breeze that clears the air and activates the life force. As a *luo*-connecting point, it brings the two Liver Officials into harmonious relationship, allowing the Gall Bladder to act as "engineer or foreman" and get on with the job of manifesting the Liver's overarching plan. In this way, processes move along in a timely way rather than lingering past their due date. The emotions flow smoothly, the vision is clear and there's hope again for the future.

The character *li* 蠡 is a complex combination of radicals. Below, we find *chong* 虫, meaning worm or insect. Above, we find *tuan* 彖, meaning hedgehog! *Li* refers to insects that, like hedgehogs, bore into and underneath things, lice, ants and other creepy things that nip and bite and energetically transform organic matter.

Gou 溝 refers to a ditch, gulley, trench, channel or ravine— any indentation through which water moves and drains. It also describes the narrow depression between the crest of the tibia and the gastrocnemius muscle, which is the anatomical location of the point. The graphic combines *shui* 氵 water with the phonetic *gou* 冓, which is described variously as the timber frames of a house under construction, a network or a pair of fish face-to-face, all implying a joining or coming together of parts.

The name tells us that this point activates, spreads and regulates the qi. It penetrates stagnation and rigidity and supports the construction of viable networks of flow. Like the strenuous activity of insects in spring or water rushing through a ditch, needling Insect Ditch - *Li Gou* gets things moving so that the work of creation can continue in a vigorous but free-flowing fashion. This is a point that says, "Clear the way! Let's go! Get on with it!" It's Spring!

Suggested Essential Oil: Blue Tansy

Blue tansy is one of the less well-known oils but one I use often in my practice. Just as tansy flowers have been traditionally used to repel ants and insects in the home, I use this essential oil to clear and repel invasive pathogens and "bugs" on the level of psyche and spirit. It has a clearing, detoxifying and ultimately stabilizing effect on the *shen* and the *hun*. In addition, it releases nervous tension, lifts the mood and has anti-inflammatory and anti-itching properties (so consider it in diluted form for bug bites!).

A drop of blue tansy can be applied directly to Insect Ditch - *Li Gou*, or dilute a few drops in a carrier oil and massage deeply along the lower ridge of the tibia to activate qi movement through the point and more radical detoxification of the Liver. The magic of this flower is that its cheerful yellow buds yield a fragrant deep-blue oil when steam distilled.

Liver 8 - Crooked Spring - *Qu Quan*
曲泉

When least expected,
I hear the song of water
beneath melting snow.

I follow the tracks of deer in the snow to a clearing in a birch grove. The snow is melting and a spring bubbles up from the dark ground. Cold. Fresh. Clear. I stand still for a while, listening to this music.

Liver 8 - Crooked Spring - *Qu Quan* 曲泉 sings the song of the waters that seep up from the lower zones of saturation, through the thawing earth in spring. It is the *he*-sea point, a hidden place at the crook of the knee, where the qi percolates deeply, down into the body to unite with the rivers and seas of the source. It has the special ability to drain off fluids when there is dampness and receive moisture and nourishment when desiccation and deficiency are present.

As a *he*-sea point, Crooked Spring - *Qu Quan* is less known for its effects on its own channel than for its ameliorating effects on diseases of the Stomach, including disordered digestion and diarrhea. In addition, it is recognized for its ability to benefit the urogenital system and drain dampness, particularly the damp heat from the Liver that may settle in the lower *jiao*, the space between the umbilicus and pelvic bone.

However, like other *he*-sea points, it can also be used to harmonize the flowing of the qi and the righteous movement of Blood in the meridians. Here is where I find this point's special medicine. In addition to its *he*-sea function, it is the Water in the Wood point on the Liver meridian, so it also brings the moistening, renewing and nourishing potency of the Water Element to the Wood. Just as winter rain and snow seep down into the soil to soften the seed and activate the upward surging thrust of the green sprout, the Water aspect of this point brings abundance, easeful flow and surging vitality to the Liver blood. This, in turn, brings grace, wellbeing and appropriate vigor to a person's emotions and actions.

I turn to this point when Wood has run out of resources. This can be because of loss of blood due to menstruation or childbirth, poor nutrition, chronic stress and emotional constraint or a constitutional tendency to Liver blood deficiency. No matter the cause, when the Wood is dry and the blood is scanty, the Liver Official becomes erratic and brittle. The ensuing state is one of either frantic anxiety and pushing or wilting exhaustion. The person loses hope and cannot see a positive future or make a realistic plan.

The point name Crooked Spring - *Qu Quan* hints at the special spirit aspect of the point. The name combines the radical *quan* 泉 spring with *qu* 曲, which is described as a bent piece of wood on a frame and refers to something crooked or curved. But *qu* 曲 can also be seen as a maze or weaving of streams that we can follow to a central gathering place. So, in a sense, the character describes the movement of water as it percolates its winding way up and down through the soil. And here is where the surprise is hidden. *Qu* 曲 also means song, a melody or winding path of notes that unite to form a piece of music. When we touch Crooked Spring - *Qu Quan*, we are inviting a person to listen to the melody of the spring that flows within them.

Suggested Treatment Strategy: Percolating the Qi

Unlike some of the points on the Gall Bladder meridian that require the assertive intentionality of the majestic warrior to activate them, I have found that Crooked Spring - *Qu Quan* responds to a subtler stimulation. When I approach this point, I feel myself entering a tender, yin and hidden space, as if following deer tracks in the forest. Insertion is deep yet gentle and unforced. Once I find the spring, I leave the point in place for a while, inviting the magic of the Water's wisdom in the Wood to do what's needed. The point can take some time to complete its work, but as a patient once said after experiencing the effect of Crooked Spring - *Qu Quan*, "As I lay there, I felt as if my whole body was being bathed in sea foam." For blood deficiency or cold dampness, five to seven rice grain moxa can be a welcome addition to the treatment.

Liver 13 - Chapter Gate - *Zhang Men*

章門

Pink moon in the west
drapes the newly budding maples
in pale mists of fire.

This morning I heard the unmistakable trill of red-winged blackbirds swarming in the swamp maples outside my bedroom window. Summer residents here in Maine, they are back early. Anxious thoughts whisper at my back: "Why are they back so soon? Can it be global warming? Will they survive if the temperatures dip below freezing again?" But, for one sweet moment of this April day, I don't care. I surrender to the chorus of joy and welcome in the spring, as the birds gorge on the first plump rosy leaf buds and celebrate their victorious return to the marsh.

Then I take a look at the morning news. More disheartening headlines. Winter temperatures in the Arctic spiked 35 degrees above the historical average. Sea ice has dropped to its lowest level on record. The latest solution on offer is climate engineering, aerosol spraying the clouds to make them more reflective. Once again, I feel myself falling into a familiar rut of hopelessness and rage.

If, as the sage Lao Tzu says, "the great truth of nature is Tao," how do I know the way of Tao when the natural world is spinning into chaos? If "one who lives in accordance with nature does not go against the way of things,"[30] how do I follow the way of things when clumsy human fingers are attempting to reweave the intricate patterns of the Divine? I resist the pull of despair as I consider Lao Tzu's counsel further. "The inner is the foundation of the outer...have faith. Follow your own shining. Be aware of your own awareness. On the darkest nights you will not stumble."[31] I take a deep breath.

I remember a message once sent to me by my friend and mentor, the Zen monk and Vietnam veteran Claude AnShin Thomas. "In Buddhism," he wrote, "it is said that 'our work is to do whatever we can to interrupt the cycles of suffering.' To this, I add two very important words, 'in us.'"

As I remember AnShin's words, a rush of qi expands my rib cage, releasing the knot of resentment in my chest and the tangle of thoughts in my mind. The anxious whispers subside, replaced by a feeling of clarity of purpose. Our work is to end the cycles of suffering and that work begins with my own awareness, right here, right now. In me.

On this early spring morning, AnShin's words are like a needle, returning me to my Tao, restoring a vision of possibility, rekindling my capacity to hope and to believe that, against all odds, there is always something I can do to make a difference. And that something starts within me.

Liver 13 - Chapter Gate - *Zhang Men* 章門 is a point for this kind of spring morning. It is a point to turn to when a person is ready to look within and open to a new possibility. It is a point to call on when it's time to complete a cycle of suffering and move on to the next chapter. Activating Chapter Gate - *Zhang Men* relaxes constraint in the diaphragm. In this way, it initiates a release of long-held breath and, when a person is ready, facilitates a deep reach into the emotional body. As the diaphragm relaxes, the qi flows more freely between the *shen* and the *hun*, allowing the guiding light of spirit to come back into connection with the soul. Free flow returns to the subtle body and habitually held resentments, anxieties and anger can be re-evaluated and transformed. By helping us to relinquish old, restrictive thoughts and chronic holding patterns, Chapter Gate - *Zhang Men* prepares us to expand

and receive the vision and hopefulness offered by its partner point, Liver 14 - Gate of Hope - *Qi Men*.

As the front-*mu* or gathering point of the Spleen, Chapter Gate - *Zhang Men* is recognized for its ability to harmonize the energies of Earth and Wood. I discover that the significance of the relationship between the Liver and Spleen is affirmed by the etymology of the point name. The character *zhang* 章 is translated as chapter or section but also can mean seal or stamp. It indicates a marking or closing of a period of time, the completion of a document, cycle or process. The character combines *yin* 音, meaning sound or musical note—立 a flute on top and 曰 a mouth below—with *shi* 十, meaning ten. The composite character indicates the completion of the chapter of a verse or a selection of music. The fact that the radical *yin* 音 is also found in the character *yi* 意 intention—the spirit of the Spleen—reinforces the idea that the Wood Element's best-laid plans, finest visions or well-wrought documents will remain incomplete and fruitless fantasies unless the Spleen and the *yi* have the strength and persistent intention to bring them down to Earth, make them real and play their music out into the world.

Opening Chapter Gate - *Zhang Men* can help Liver qi to flow and grow more freely, thus resolving stagnation and allowing for the completion of an organic process or a chapter in our lives. I consider this point when the Wood is ready to let go and move forward. I have found it helpful for physical symptoms such as abdominal distension and impaired digestion and psychological symptoms such as smoldering resentments and hopelessness.

As the Chapter Gate swings open, Liver qi travels gracefully across the K'o cycle and the diaphragm to nourish the Spleen. In this way, the grandparent, Wood, delivers its precious legacy to its grandchild, Earth. Through the Liver's gifts of vision, clarity and direction, the Spleen's capacity for conviction, strength and generosity is renewed, and the hopeful possibilities of spring can become real, even in uncertain times.

Liver 14 - Gate of Hope - *Qi Men*
期 門

Gathering moonlight
for their breakfast, clouds at dawn
spill dew drops on my hair.

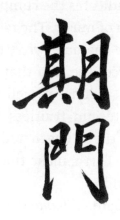

I open the door and see that it is spring. The world is once again miraculously renewed. A tiny seed of faith sprouts green in my heart. I step outside to begin another day of healing—for myself, for other beings, for the world. Liver 14 - Gate of Hope - *Qi Men* 期 門 is a master point for the Spring season—a point of new, green vision, of liberation and renewal.

The name of the point is composed of two characters. The character on the left, *qi* 期, combines *yue* 月, the picture of the moon, with the phonetic *qi* 其, a picture of a sieve or a winnowing basket on a stand. The moon refers to the passage of time through the lunar phases: from month to month, season to season, year to year. The sieve or winnowing basket refers to a process of gathering, specifically the gathering of what is needed and letting go of what is not. Winnowing involves throwing the unsorted products of harvest into the air so that the wind blows away the lighter chaff, while the heavier grains fall back down for recovery. The inference here is that this point allows us to gather the wisdom of time, to carry forward what we need and let go of what we don't in order to move into a new season.

The character on the right, *men* 門, is a picture of the two doors of a gate. Together, the characters that form the point name *Qi Men* 期 門 tell us that when we needle this point, we are opening the twin gates of the rib cage and freeing up the flow of our breath and life force. With the winds of exhalation, I let go of the chaff, and with the inhalation, I take in the energies I need to move forward.

As the exit point of the Liver meridian, Gate of Hope - *Qi Men* supports the smooth flow of qi between the Liver and the Lungs. I call on this point when the Liver pulse is abundant and strong and the Lung pulse is weak. Opening this gate when the conditions are right allows the qi to rise from the Liver to the Lungs, ending and beginning a full cycle of the life force through the meridians. The Liver relaxes and the Lungs expand, the marriage of the *hun* and *po* is renewed and the vision of Wood illuminates the inspirations of Metal. As the Wood Element is freed to deliver its gifts to the soul, the blessings of joy, humor and hope return to the Heart space just as green vitality returns to the world after a long, cold winter.

I think of Chapter Gate - *Zhang Men* and Liver 14 - Gate of Hope - *Qi Men* as soul gates. They act as conduits that open communication between the *hun, yi* and *po*. As my body and breath souls align with my intention, I feel the flow of the Tao move through me. And then, as a patient once said after I needled these points, "I feel like my body is coming back to life in spring after a very long winter."

Suggested Essential Oil: Bergamot

We can move qi through Gate of Hope - *Qi Men* with a needle, a touch or an appropriately placed word. However, I have found that the point is particularly responsive to essential oils. These oils must be of high quality and free from rancidity. In my practice, I often turn to bergamot, which has a gentle yet powerful effect on this point. A drop or two of this potent, qi-moving oil on Gate of Hope - *Qi Men* relaxes and smooths the energies of the Liver and Wood Element as it relieves feelings of tension, irritability, resentment and hopelessness.

In situations where there is significant holding in the diaphragm, I dilute a few drops of high-grade bergamot essential oil with a cold-pressed carrier oil such as almond or avocado. I go for just enough bergamot in the carrier oil so the aroma is discernable. This is especially good for patients with chronic tension in the diaphragm and accumulated Liver heat and stagnation.

A caveat with this oil: less is more! A drop or two is sufficient to create change. Be careful not to expose skin to immediate sunlight after application, as the oil, like the chlorophyll of new spring leaves, is photosensitive.

A note on location: Gate of Hope - *Qi Men* has two accepted locations, directly below the nipple in the sixth intercostal space or further down, directly below the nipple in a small notch at the inferior border of the rib cage. Both of these point locations are doorways that open a path of qi through the diaphragm. I suggest choosing the one that responds most to touch and pressure on any given day.

Fire: Summer Season

The *I Ching* speaks of Fire as a paradox, something bright that has darkness at its core, something that rises toward Heaven yet is tethered to the Earth, something formless that requires form to nourish it. The text reminds us that "everything that gives light is dependent on something to which it clings, in order that it may continue to shine."[1] Fire's characteristic flickering, up-and-down flame reflects the *enantiodromia*, the paradoxical dynamic, that defines its nature. Its yang luminosity, activity and heat are dependent on its relationship to a dark, quiescent opposite, the yin matter that nourishes it. This paradox is the secret of Fire's flickering dance and its ever-shifting radiance.

The Chinese character for Fire is *huo* 火. In the graphic, we can see a fire with dancing flames. The extensive, upward, downward, inward, flickering nature of the Element is deftly expressed by the four simple lines of the character.

The Fire Element is related to the season of Summer, the time of year when the solar forces of heat, light and growth are at their most exuberant. We find Fire at the very peak of the Five Element Wheel, at the point closest to Heaven, the most yang, negentropic position of the circle. This placement reminds us of Fire's tendency to rise but also of the inevitability of the subsequent fall. Ultimately, even Fire cannot resist the downward, entropic pull of Earth's gravity and the limitations of the material world.

Kigo words evoke the joyous yet ephemeral atmosphere of summer. Waking early to dawn infused with the fragrance of peony blossoms. Wild iris at the cool edge of the marsh and the blue heron dipping her long bill into the water in search of fish. Heat lightning and rolling thunder, a sudden shower of summer rain. Warm sunlight ripening tiny strawberries in the grassy meadow. Tree frogs at twilight and fireflies in the night. Stars falling in the moonlit pond. Fire calls us to reveal our true nature, to open to the unbearable beauty of creation, to risk the heartbreak of loss in order to love the world more deeply.

Vegetative Expression

The energetic of this Element is expressed by the blossoming flower lifted skyward by its innate desire to be admired, enjoyed, pollinated and touched by the light of Heaven. Yet, at the very moment that the bud opens to receive the full force of the sunlight, the petals are overtaken by the constraints of weight and form. They cannot stay star-bound and before long will drop one by one from the green stem to the ground below. The blossom's seductive beauty, elegant yet fragile structure, indomitable spirit and anti-gravitational expansive nature tell us a great deal about the Fire Element as it lives within our own souls.[2]

This moment of blossoming, this fleeting moment of high Summer, arrives with a sudden surprising clamor of color and then, almost before we catch a glimpse of the ecstatic beauty, softens and fades under the influence of the yin. The petals fall and the ovule of the flower begins to grow heavy and swell to form the seeds and fruits that become the harvest of Late Summer. In the profusion of Summer's blossoms, at the peak moment of Fire's exuberant "I blossom," comes the first intimation of compassion and gracious giving, which leads to Earth's "I nourish and care for the world."

Color/Sound/Odor/Emotion

The Color of Fire is Red

The Yellow Emperor's Class of Internal Medicine says "Red is the color of the South, it pervades the heart and retains the essential substances within the heart."[3] To diagnose the health of the Fire Element, look at the sides of the eyes, temples and laugh lines around the mouth for a range of red, from cardinal feathers to rose petals to rust. "When their color is red like blood they are without life... When their color is red like a cock's comb they are full of life."[4] It is also important not to overlook the "lack of Fire" color, which is gray and looks like ashes smudged or brushed across the skin. Unlike the black or blue-black of Water, which is slow to change, the "lack of Fire" ashen gray can sometimes fill in with red when a person laughs or is touched by compassion. However, like the flickering flame, the red in a "lack of Fire" person will come and go quickly and, even after many years of treatment, may remain unstable.

The Sound is Laugh

The laugh sound may come as actual laughter, especially at inappropriate moments in a conversation, or as a hint of an upward lilt or giggle at the end of a sentence. However it's expressed, the laugh sound has a lifting energy that lightens the overall feeling of communication.

The Odor is Scorched

In balance, the scorched odor is like the smell of a hot iron on clean cotton cloth or slightly burnt toast. When out of balance, it can smell like burnt meat, the aftermath of a bonfire or overly heated sweat.

The Emotion is Joy

In health, Fire expresses as appropriately modulated warmth, happiness that easily comes and goes in response to the environment, a stable flame that flickers but is not extinguished. Out of balance, it can show up as hysteria, mania and a desperate grasping at happiness or a lack-of-joy flatness that completely dampens relatedness.

The Officials

Unlike the other four elements, which only have two officials, the Fire Element has four Officials: the Heart Official or Supreme Monarch and the three ministers in its service.

The Heart Official holds the office of the Monarch. It is the Supreme Controller of the kingdom of the body, mind and spirit. It is the sovereign ruler who governs every organ, every rhythm and every activity of being. From our first to last breath, our Hearts maintain the flow of blood in our bodies and the flow of life through our souls. Book Three of the *Neijing Suwen* emphasizes the crucial importance of the Heart Monarch:

> [W]hen the monarch is intelligent and enlightened, there is peace and contentment among his subjects...there are no more dangers and perils, the earth is considered glorious and prosperous. But when the monarch is not intelligent and enlightened, the twelve officials become dangerous and perilous; the use of Tao is obstructed and blocked and Tao no longer circulates warnings against physical excesses.[5]

J. R. Worsley writes that the Heart Official is "like an emperor who controls and co-ordinates, but his commands can only succeed as long as they accord with the wishes and desires of his people."[6] The Heart cannot "do" but must do by and through relationship and connection. Taoist healers understood that the successful Monarch accomplishes its Herculean tasks effortlessly, by simply being centered at the center. When the kingdom is functioning well, the Monarch controls every aspect of the body, mind and spirit through the wisdom of *wu wei* 無 為, doing by not doing. As the Taoist sage Lao Tzu writes, "The highest type of ruler is one whose existence the people are barely aware of."[7]

The classical texts emphasize that the Heart must be empty in order to fulfill its crucial function, which is to be the residence or throne room of the *shen*, the spirit of the Fire Element that Taoists recognized as the Divine spark of conscious awareness. The Heart must be empty in order to be filled. Claude Larre expresses this paradox by saying, "The heart is essentially void because the void is the only possible dwelling place for the spirits."[8] It is this *wu*—this emptiness—that must be diligently protected so that the *shen*, the Divine light of the self, the true radiance of Heavenly Fire, can illuminate our way along the path of Tao.

The empty space at the center of the Heart is the residence of the *shen*, the Divine seed of starlight that comes to us from Heaven at the moment of our conception and that gives us the capacity to know ourselves, to "see" our way and to shine the light of our own unique self—our own divinity—out into the world. For alchemists throughout space and time, this spark of divinity is the "true gold." For the Taoists, it was considered the most precious, the most potent, yet also the most vulnerable, aspect of our being.

The *shen* is the light that comes down from Heaven to shine through us. It is the organizing light of consciousness and it holds the seed spark of our destiny within it. From this perspective, the critical need for the organism to protect the spark of the *shen* becomes clear, and we can view the three Fire Officials as the guardians at the gate of the chamber of the Divine. But we can also understand them as aspects of our psychological boundaries, the lines of protection we open and close as we engage in our relationships and Heart connection with ourselves, with others and to the cosmos.

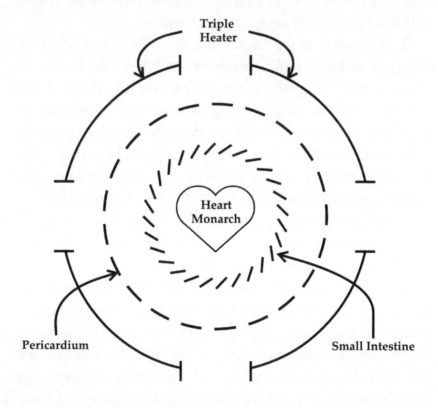

KINGDOM OF THE HEART

I imagine the Heart and the three other Fire Officials as living together side by side within the palace of the upper mansion.

They are separate yet interrelated. Each one has its own unique and crucial protective function on the level of emotions and relationships, yet one without the others cannot do the job well.

Triple Heater

I think of the Triple Heater as the most yang of the four Fire Officials. The Triple Heater meridian runs up the protective back side of the arm. In the imaginary castle of the self, he stands at the Outer Frontier Gate as keeper of the moat, protector of the palace and manager of the drawbridge. The *Neijing Suwen* tells us that this official "plans the construction of ditches and sluices, and creates waterways."[9] He is the emissary of the emperor stationed at the nation's borders, "responsible for opening up the passages and irrigation. The regulation of fluids stem from it"[10] and for maintaining "the balance between inside and outside."[11] Everything the Heart needs for the smooth regulation of the kingdom must enter through this gate and everything the Heart needs to communicate outward exits through it. The Triple Heater allows us to spread our warmth out into the world and to receive the warmth from our environment. In this way, the Triple Heater regulates the temperature of our Fire on physical, emotional and spiritual levels.

Psychological symptoms specifically associated with this official are often related to managing connections between our inner and outer worlds. When I experience difficulties putting myself out into the world, receiving the supplies I need from others, knowing how to regulate the warmth of intimacy or simply having an enjoyable time at a gathering, I know that this official is asking for support. Conversely, a

Triple Heater imbalance can manifest as excess engagement with the outer world and inability to access inner resources.

The critical question that the Triple Heater asks is: in or out? Is this person, idea, experience, opportunity worthy of crossing the drawbridge and coming closer into my Heart? Will it support the wellbeing of the kingdom or will it drain reserves and toxify the environment? And if I choose to walk across the Outer Frontier Gate to make contact with another being, what do I actually need to know, carry and do in order to protect myself wisely?

Pericardium

Blood sibling to the Triple Heater, the Pericardium is like an envelope or woven matrix that protects the Heart and acts as a more intimate yin guardian to the Monarch. The Pericardium meridian runs from the nipple of the breast down the protective back side of the arm and, in the imaginary castle of the self, she is the guardian at the door of the inner frontier. I think of this official as a ruby-colored energy shield or semi-permeable membrane that surrounds and protects the Heart. This official functions as a membrane that opens for the passage of love and warmth and other energies that support and vitalize the Monarch, and yet effortlessly closes when negative energies approach. It can be likened to a maternal womb that nourishes, protects and maintains the wellbeing of a Divine fetus that is the spark of spirit at the center of our being.[12]

The Pericardium brings her peculiarly yin strengths to bear on her work as the Monarch's bodyguard through her sensitivity, malleability, resilience, determination and fierceness. This valiant spiritual warrior gracefully wards off blows aimed at the Heart. She regulates arterial and venous circulation and sexual secretions on a physical level and trust and intimacy on a psychological level. The smooth functioning of this official allows me to feel a sense of safety in relationships, trust and openness to others and to myself. Common psychological symptoms I see in myself and in patients in my practice include being overly porous to the feelings and vibrations of others and prematurely open to intimacy. In these situations, the Pericardium Official has lost her ability to know when to close the door to the inner chamber. Through trauma or repeated emotional invasion, her protective shield is fixed in an excessively permeable "stuck open" state. On the other hand, an imbalance at this level can lead to an overly closed membrane that leaves the Heart feeling cut off and alone, unable to make deep, safe and lasting connections.

The question that the Pericardium asks is: yes or no? In the case of the Heart Protector, it is critical to remember that, when the answer is "No!," "No!" is a full sentence. The Pericardium Official asks: is this person, idea, experience or opportunity worthy of my time, attention and intimate consideration? Will it support me in living my Tao if I say "yes" to this person, experience or idea and invite them to come closer into my Heart? Will it support the wellbeing of the kingdom and the self or will it threaten my integrity, inject toxicity into my inner environment? And if I choose to open the inner frontier gate in order to make contact with another being, what do I actually need to know, carry and do in order to protect myself wisely?

The Small Intestine

The Small Intestine Official holds the office of Separator of Pure from Impure. He is a yang official whose job is to scrupulously guard the doorway to the Monarch's chamber. This official "is responsible for receiving and making things thrive. Transformed substances stem from it."[13] Like a trusted communication minister for the Queen, he must listen intently in order to separate the pure from impure and discern what does and does not belong in the Monarch's chamber. The Small Intestine meridian runs along the lateral side of the arm. I think of it as a kind of knife-edge that can cut through the dross in order to distill the essences. I picture him as a minister of the mail who is responsible for sorting through and refining every piece of information, every request and every communication that attempts to reach the Monarch. It is up to the Small Intestine to discern what will support the Heart's integrity and wellbeing and what will not. In the end, he decides what and who is pure, nourishing and refined enough to enter the inner sanctum, be integrated and ultimately become part of the Monarch of the Self. And in the end, it is he who decides who and what is "not me" and needs to be filtered out of the system.

This official's task is to sort out the pure fine essences that will nourish and support the Heart and to send the impure substances down to the Large Intestine for excretion. Listening carefully, culling out what is true and necessary and then letting the rest go is accomplished effortlessly by a healthy Small Intestine Official. On a psychological level, I recognize a troubled Small Intestine Official when I meet a patient who has no ability to discern what they need or who cannot benefit from the nutrients they absorb, whether on a physical, psychological or spiritual level. A troubled Small Intestine is unable to help the Heart to distinguish self from other, good from evil, healthy relationships or information from toxic. Most importantly, a disturbance at the level interferes with my capacity to know myself and to hear the wisdom of my own Heart.

The Small Intestine asks and answers the question: is this

me or you? Is this person, idea, experience or opportunity worthy of being taken into my Heart, absorbed and integrated into the wholeness of my self? Is it adequately refined and clear or is it still mixed with toxins or undigested waste that will confuse or dim the light of the Monarch? If I choose to invite and absorb this person, value, idea or experience directly into my Heart, my self and my identity, what do I actually need to know, carry and do in order to protect myself wisely?

The Heart

The Heart of Supreme Controller is said to be the "minister of the monarch who excels through insight and understanding." This official "hold[s] the office of Lord and Sovereign. The radiance of the spirits stems from it."[14] Although the Heart is the most protected, most interior of all the officials and considered yin, it also has a yang aspect. Through its contraction and expansion, the Heart is able to resolve paradoxes and bring together opposites to form a new whole. The Heart begins to beat a brief 22 days after conception and continues to beat without rest until the moment of death. In order to carry out its role as sovereign and ceaseless keeper of the rhythm of life, the void at the center of the Heart must be protected so that the *shen* has a proper home. It does this through special wisdom of *wu wei*, doing by not doing. Psychological symptoms that arise when the *shen* is not adequately protected and well rooted in the Heart include disassociation from self, muddled thinking and communication and depression or lack of integrity to life and relationships.

The Heart asks and also answers the question: *wu* or *wei*? To do or not do? Or simply to be? When is yang action, penetration and initiation most in accordance with my

Tao? And when is yin receptivity, gestation and non-doing the most skillful response? When to expand and when to contract. And, most of all, when to clear the Monarch's chamber of all thoughts, worries and emotions. When to do nothing but put my two hands together, touch Spirit Gate to Spirit Gate in prayer and open to the light of the Divine within me.

Shen: The Spirit of Fire

The spirit of the Fire Element is the *shen* 神, translated as spirit or divinity. In the mythical language of ancient Chinese embryology, it is said that the *shen* is a speck of Divine light that comes to us directly from the stars. At the moment of conception, the scoop of the Big Dipper ladles up starlight from the Milky Way and pours it down into the mother's womb. This starlight enters the developing embryo through the primary cell division that eventually centers at a point at the top of the head, Governing Vessel 20 - One Hundred Meetings - *Bai Hui*. Within moments, the *shen* begins to organize the unfolding growth of the person. At the moment of death, when its task is complete, it is liberated from the body, exits through One Hundred Meetings - *Bai Hui* and returns to its natural home in the Heavens.

The character for *shen* is made up of two parts. The radical on the left *shih* 礻 is a picture of an altar. It means "to divine" or "influences coming down from above." *Shih* 礻 has a pictorial and semantic relationship to lightning; like lightning, it refers to yang fiery influences from above that illuminate or ignite the world below.

The phonetic radical on the right *shen* 申 is a picture of two hands grasping a rope. It means to extend or expand and, specifically, to forge a connection between Above and Below. From the etymology of the character and the associated myth, we come to understand *shen* as the Divine spirit that gives the Heavenly orders that precipitate life and organize the unfolding of our earthly being. *Shen* activates and ignites the unfolding of our being but also gives us the mandate for our life purpose and is the guiding light of destiny.

Throughout our life, the *shen* organizes and maintains the integrity of the self. By day it shines outward and can be seen as the sparkle in the eyes of a healthy human being. At night, it drops down to rest in the Heart and helps the *hun* to weave the messages of dreams. By day and by night, it illuminates and guides us along the path of Tao. At the moment of death, the *shen* rises back to Heaven through the point at the top of the head and returns to its home in the stars. The coming and going of the *shen* mark the beginning and end of our unique, individual, embodied presences in the world.

The *shen* functions as the director of *wu shen*, the five spirits, as a whole. In this way, we can say that it presides over and organizes awareness on all levels. On its own, we consider it the spirit of enlightened insight and conscious awareness. It endows us with the capacity to know our self and to communicate the needs, knowledge and wisdom of the self to others with whom we come into contact. Through this capacity to relate to self and others, the *shen* allows us to know and express our authentic nature and to walk the path of our own Tao. When the function of the *shen* is interrupted, anxiety, panic, insomnia, muddled thinking and depression may result. But beyond these specific troubling symptoms, there is the sense that the true self is absent and the person's life lacks purpose and meaning. The light of spirit has been extinguished from the lantern of their being.

In the sacred mountain that is the symbol of the self, the

shen resides on the peak, high above the treeline, close to the sun, moon and stars of Heaven. The pure consciousness that is the light of the *shen* can be blinding to our ordinary eyes. This is why we need the *hun* soul to add a bit of yin to its dazzling Fire. Then, with the help of our dreams and the Heart open and attentive, "the spirit is suddenly revealed through one's own consciousness...as though the wind has blown away the cloud."[15]

Fire's spirit question: How am I expressing my true self in my life and in my relationships?

Spirit Animal: The Red Bird

The spirit of the Heart resembles a Red Bird. Its spirit name is Origin of the Cinnabar Field and its given name is To Preserve the *Shen*. The Red Bird comes and goes from our Hearts through an opening at the center of the chest just below Conception Vessel 15 - Dove Tail - *Jiu Wei*. The Chinese character for Red Bird is *zhu jiao* 朱 鷦.

While *zhu* does mean red, it's not an ordinary red. *Zhu* refers to the color of cedar, specifically the trunk of the cedar tree, known for its deep red core or "heart," and its longevity and resistance to deterioration. The color of the cedar tree's core is burnished rust, close to the color of blood and also close to the color of the alchemical metal cinnabar. Cinnabar is formed when cool mercury and hot sulfur are heated and combined.[16] Taoist alchemists prize cinnabar as an expression of the alchemical marriage, a resolution of the paradox of yin and yang through the creation of a new substance. The color tells us something about the Red Bird's magic as well as the Heart's ability to resolve seemingly irresolvable paradoxes.

Zhu jiao is not a normal bird. Its name in Chinese is specific and intentional. *Jiao* refers to a little bird, a sparrow or wren, a bird that prefers to nest and forage close to people rather than alone in the forest. It is a sociable, familiar bird, a bird that wants to relate to us, to live alongside us and be part of our daily experience. Sparrows and wrens are ordinarily plain brown and easily overlooked, but *zhu jiao* is special. It is cinnabar red, red the color of our own blood. Unlike an ordinary bird, the Red Bird is attracted to fire and loves heat. When it sees fire, *zhu jiao* shakes its feathers and flies up to Heaven. As it rises, it becomes a dragon. As it climbs higher, it becomes a tiger. As it flies even higher, it does not disappear but becomes a four-star constellation in the southern sky. Later, when the Red Bird returns to its familiar nest, it brings the messages of dragons, tigers and stars "down to earth" and into our everyday life.

Alchemical texts sometimes describe the Heart as a hanging lotus flower that is able to change Water into blood. From this, we know that the Heart's spiritual task is to transform the Water of ordinary life experience into something mythical, something rich and nourishing, a kind of blood that is necessary not only to our bodies but also to our souls. The gift of the Red Bird is the gift of Fire. Like Fire, it has a cheerful, friendly intimacy that transforms when necessary into a wild, courageous fierceness that preserves the spirit and allows the Heart to work its Divine alchemy.

The Red Bird is the protector of the southern direction. We call on the Red Bird to support us when we face the heat of intimacy and love, the Fire of transformation and the riotous blossoming of summer. The Red Bird flies before us as we move into a relationship, as we walk forward into the passion of creativity, as we valiantly strive to know our true nature and shine the light of our self out into the world. It clings to us like a dear friend and shields us from the unnecessary, the dangerous, the unforgiving and the crass. And when it opens its red wings wide to protect our Hearts, the darkness slips off its feathers like summer rain.

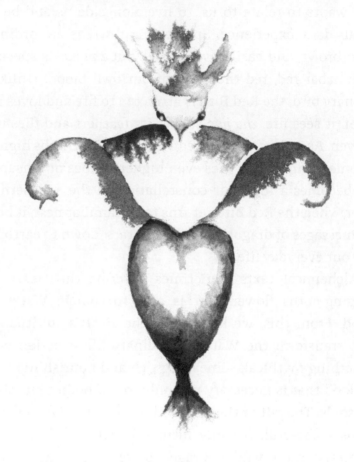

RED BIRD

Archetype: *Connunctio/Nigredo* or The Marriage of Opposites

The union, dissolution and reunion of opposites form the foundational dynamic of all alchemical systems. Whether we are working with the ebb and flow of yin and yang in organic life, the melding of sulfur and mercury in the alchemical laboratory, the interplay of sun and moon, light and dark, masculine and feminine, or the rhythmic pulsation of connection and disconnection in human relationships, we are encountering the creative mystery of the cosmos.

In Taoist alchemy, it is understood that the primal opposites of yin and yang emerge directly from the undifferentiated wholeness of Tao. These two original parents bring forth the entire macrocosmic universe and their interplay continues to unfold through every microcosmic aspect of creation. Their connection is life and their dissolution is death. Ultimately, at the end of time, they, along with all phenomena, return again to the archaic chaos of Tao.

In Taoist philosophy, this primal dance of opposites is called the *tai ji* 太 极 Supreme Ultimate. It is represented by the yin/yang symbol, the two fish chasing each other's tails.

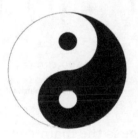

TAI JI - YIN/YANG SYMBOL

In European alchemy, where the goal of inner work became less focused on the spiritual development of the sage through internal practices and more on the incarnation of the soul through relationships, the creative dance of opposites was called the *Connunctio* or Sacred Marriage. The *Connunctio* is represented by two lovers, the Alchemical King and Queen. Its most widely recognized symbol is the eclipse, the marriage of Sol and Luna, the sacred union of sun and moon.

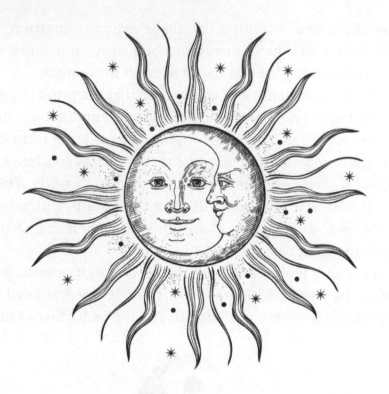

SOL AND LUNA

Source: Natalia Krechetova

This celestial marriage is the main concern of one of the primary medieval alchemical texts, *The Rosary of the Philosophers*, where we read:

> I am Luna, increasing moist and cold, and you are Sol, hot and moist. When we shall be coupled in equity of state in a mansion which is not made otherwise but with light fire, having with itself great heat in which we shall be emptied, and we shall be as a woman that wants the fruit of her increase... Then we shall rejoice and be exalted in the exultation of the spirit... Then the lamp of your light will be poured into my lamp, and of you and of me there will be a mixture, as of wine and sweet water...[17]

The *Connunctio* is the embodied expression of the principle of synergy—two or more parts coming together to create a field of potential from which a third new possibility can be born. This vibrating field of potential is present whenever opposites come into contact, whether the opposites are two atoms of different natures, two elements, two ideas or two people. In Taoist alchemy, the third that is born from the interplay of yang and yin is qi—the vital energy of life itself. In the Western tradition, it is represented by the archetype of the "Divine Child."

The Divine Child is "the third," the new life that is born of the *Connunctio*. It is the alchemical counterpart and soul expression of the physical child that is born of sexual union between a woman and a man. The Divine Child is the new idea, the original work of art, the surprising solution, the unexpected connection to self that is the product of our relationship to our own Heart and our devoted inner work. It is the wisdom, insight, compassion and expansion of self that is engendered through the challenging dance of committed outer relationship over time. Of the child, C. G. Jung writes in *The Archetypes of the Collective Unconscious*:

> [T]he child paves the way for a future change of personality. In the individuation process, it anticipates the figure that comes from the synthesis of conscious and unconscious elements in the personality...a symbol which unites the opposites; a mediator, bringer of healing, that is, one who makes whole...[18]

The Divine Marriage refers to the art and craft of *eros*, creative connection and vital relationship. In their regal copulation, the two Heavenly lights, the sun and moon, bring together the opposites of gold and silver, light and dark, hot and cold, masculine and feminine to create enduring illumination—the philosopher's stone or what is recognized in the European alchemical tradition as the incarnate soul. The *Connunctio* is the celebration of this vibrant creativity. The exuberant atmosphere of the *Connunctio* is in the background of every love affair, every wedding, every flower that opens its petals to the sun. This lifting of the Heart and joyful attitude is the natural response of our being to the negentropic movement toward love, blossoming, expansion and illumination that are the hallmarks of the Fire Element.

However, it's crucial to understand that the *Connunctio* also has its own *enantiodromia*, its own innate tendency to transform into its opposite once it has reached its fullest expression. At the nadir of the yin, there is an implicit tendency for the yang to irrupt, and at the apex of yang, the yin emerges. With every marriage, with every celebration of connection and creativity, with every birth, with every illumination, an opposite arises. In fairy tales, this opposite is represented by the forgotten 13th fairy that shows up with a curse at the celebratory feast of the newborn princess. In the creative process, it is the inevitable self-doubt and critical voices that attack after a time of rich productivity. In new love, it is the first argument. It is postpartum depression, the setting of the sun, the waning of the full moon, the tipping back down of the *sheng* cycle at the height of Summer.

In medieval alchemical art, alongside richly colored paintings of celestial weddings, we discover pictures of burning cities charred to smoking ruins, bloodthirsty lions devouring the sun, couples attacking each other tooth and claw, kings beheaded and thrown to dogs. These images point to an alchemical understanding of the necessity and inevitability of dissolution after union. European alchemists referred to this disruption of connection and its accompanying states of despair, grief and rage as the *Nigredo* or darkening. They recognized it as absolutely essential to the opus, the great work of spiritual transformation.

The *Nigredo* is a necessary part of the alchemical process. It arises out of the resistance of yang spirit to its earthly fall. The *Nigredo* is the spirit's encounter with the downward pull of gravity, with the limitations of material existence, the restricting boundaries of time and space and the inevitability of aging and corruption. The *Nigredo* is an inevitable reality that cannot be eradicated, but with consciousness, it can be worked with and transformed. Buried in the *Nigredo*'s dark shadow, there is hidden gold. Through our conscious acceptance of the *Nigredo* and our willingness to bear its slow and painful wearing down of illusion, the light of the spirit is incarnated and integrated in a real way into our everyday life.

As with the flickering yang flame that clings to its nourishing yin fuel in order to maintain its brightness, the *Connunctio* must cling to the *Nigredo* and learn to love its darkness. Only in this way can Fire persevere, hold steady and enter into the realm of time and space. Only in this way can spirit be embodied and the Sacred Marriage of the soul be realized.

Alchemy: Opening the Heart

The *shen* comes to us from the stars at the moment of conception. During our lives, this speck of starlight resides in the Heart. It illuminates our destiny and true nature, guides us along the path of Tao and, at the end of the journey, it leads our spirit back to the infinite sky realms of Heaven. It is said that the bowl of the Heart must be open at the top in order to receive the radiance of the *shen*, the Divine influences that come to us from above.

The Chinese character for Heart, *xin*, is a picture of a bowl with three lines. The lines on either side are said to be a primitive representation of the main veins and arteries. If we look at the character, we can see the opening at the top of the bowl and the speck of *shen* resting at the center.

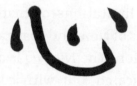

XIN - HEART

The Taoist alchemical text, the *Xiuzhen Tu* (The Chart of the Cultivation of Ultimate Reality), tells us that the Heart has openings that allow the spirit to enter.[19] These openings also act as conduits, pathways that connect a human life to *wu*, the undifferentiated emptiness of Tao. The more open the Heart, the more the person is illuminated by spirit and the more open to the swirling, fertile chaos that is Tao. The text goes further to say that in the middle of the Heart of a very wise man, there are seven openings. In the Heart of a person of middle knowledge, there are five. And in the case of persons with little knowledge, "the Heart has no openings at all, the undifferentiated emptiness of *wu* and the light of Heaven cannot penetrate into their being."[20] Without these openings in our Heart, we cannot become truly human and our soul withers, unnourished by the Divine.

The 13th-century Persian poet Jalal ad-Din Muhammad Rumi tells us something similar when he says, "Love comes with a knife, not some shy question...don't put blankets over the drum! Open completely."[21]And then, "Imagine the time when the particle you are returns where it came from! The family darling comes home. Wine, without being contained in cups is handed around."[22]

The wisdom of the Heart teaches us to celebrate the process of being broken open, to not shut down to ecstasy and the inevitable losses and betrayals of love, but rather to learn to bear the emotional heat that is the transformational agent of the soul. The blossoming of the Heart requires the cracking open of the seed and the acceptance of the flower's falling petals.

This is the paradox of the Fire that only the Heart can resolve: that in opening to love, we will experience wounding and only through this wounding can we connect to spirit and heal back into our wholeness.

Fire Spirit Points

Heart 1 - Utmost Source - *Ji Quan*
極泉

One wild rose between
two stones. A single blossom
opens to the sun.

Heart 1 - Utmost Source - *Ji Quan* 極泉 is like a hidden spring I discover in the woods after climbing up the sunny side of a mountain on a hot summer afternoon. I lean down and scoop this water up between my palms. As I pour it over my face and down the back of my neck, my Heart is calmed and my breathing settles. This stillness, this tranquility, this freedom of flow and clarity of presence...these are the spirit gifts of Utmost Source - *Ji Quan*, the summit spring, the entry point of the Heart meridian.

In Chinese medicine, the Heart is the Monarch, the organizing principle of the kingdom of the body, mind and spirit. In addition, the Heart is viewed as the residence of the *shen*, the illuminating spark of spirit that guides my individual life. The Chinese character for Heart, *xin* 心, is shaped like an open bowl, empty at the center so that the Heavenly *shen* has a safe place to rest within me. For the ancient Egyptians, the hieroglyphic for Heart was a picture of a vase, which was said to be the storehouse of memory and truth. In all traditional cultures, the Heart was understood to be a sacred center, a vessel, which needs vigilant protection and care in order for life to flourish. Archetypally, "the heart shares with the lotus flower and the rose the qualities of the hidden, enfolded center beneath the outer surface of things, the secret abode of consciousness, locked away, virgin and so inviolate that if we want to 'let someone in,' we must give them 'the key.'"[23]

Utmost Source - *Ji Quan* gives us the key to the Heart. It is the point where the qi of the Heart leaves the safe, secluded palace of the Heart and begins its journey down the arm to the fingertip and then out into the world. *Ji* 極 is a picture of *mu* 木 a tree next to *ji* 亟 a man extending himself between Heaven and Earth next to the crossed threads radical *yao* 爻 that is used to indicate mutual action and reaction, hope but also something rare and special. *Ji* means the farthest extremity of a pole, the extreme limit, reaching the utmost and highest point, the beginning, the end and the turning point.

Quan 泉 combines the radical *bai* 白 white over *shui* 水 water. It is a picture of pure, clear, vibrant spring water gushing upward from the Earth and it is translated to mean fountain, source or spring.

When I needle Utmost Source - *Ji Quan*, I feel I am tapping into the spring where the qi of the Heart is at its most plentiful, fresh and vital. When the point opens, these fine, precious, life-giving energies rise up from the depths of an inner source to nourish and replenish my body and my soul.

I consider this point when a person has lost connection to their sense of who they are. Symptoms include confusion about desires, lack of life goals or an inability to express personal needs. In addition, I have found that blockage at this point can lead to feelings of numbness, deadness, overriding exhaustion, disorientation and oppression. Intercostal tightness and pain can accompany the lack of joy symptomatic of Heart constraint and stasis, and both respond well to the liberating movement of qi that this point engenders.

Utmost Source - *Ji Quan* is, indeed, the rare and special point that I turn to when a person is "at the end of their rope." When there is dryness on any level of being, this point brings refreshing, thirst-quenching waters to the soul and to the body. It reunites us with our deepest nature and connects us to the divinity of the self. In this way, it can be said to be the spring of the life force from which the waters of our spirit flow, the sacred center where we go to be refreshed and renewed, where we recover our hope and find our way back to the truth of who we are.

Heart 7 - Spirit Gate - *Shen Men*

神門

Light as a finger
tip the breeze, ignites a fire
hidden in my heart.

At dawn, I take my cup of tea and go down to the garden. The slight mist is already burning away with the rising sun. As I look out across the field, it seems that the sky gate has opened and Heaven has showered the grass with rainbows: purple tufted cow vetch, wild blue irises, lupines, bluets, buttercups and, here and there, a first crimson splash of poppies. On this early summer morning, I feel the presence of the *shen* in the tender exuberance of the white snow-pea blossoms, the tremble and flutter of goldfinches in the maple trees, the quickening warmth of the sunlight and, most of all, the shimmer of joy that coats each leaf, each bird, each blossom and the tender edges of my Heart with a glaze of Summer Fire.

Heart 7 - Spirit Gate - *Shen Men* 神門 opens the gate for the comings and goings of the *shen*. Like early summer dawn, the point is tender yet filled with potency. When it is needled with care and clear intention at the appropriate moment, I have found it to be unparalleled in its capacity to settle scattered *shen*, restore presence, calm hyperactivity and bring a person back into connection with their own authentic nature. As a fiery patient of mine says each time I touch this point on her wrist, "That got at it. I'm back!" Then I see the star sparkle return to her eyes and the light of awareness in her face and I know that the point has done its work.

The point name is composed of two parts: *shen* 神 spirit and *men* 門 gate. *Shen* combines two radicals: *shih* 礻 with the phonetic *shen* 申. *Shih* 礻 is described as a stylized picture of an altar, but an earlier form of the character 示 shows that it is also a picture of the light rays of the sun, moon and stars shining down as three vertical lines from the sky. *Shih* is translated to mean altar but also "to divine" and "influences from above." The rays of celestial light coming down from above endow us with powers of divination, the spiritual sight that allows us to see and follow the pathway to our destiny.

Shen 申 is a picture of two hands holding a rope. It implies something that extends vertically between Heaven and Earth: a lightning bolt, a ladder, a ray of light. When I wrap my hands around this rope—whether through meditation, prayer, presence, love or wonder—I am connected to the Divine. I receive the influxes of Heaven into my Heart and allow their light to guide my actions in the world of matter. In this way, the *shen* "give us signs that help us to 'see' or 'divine' which way to go to keep to our path of Tao."[24]

This point acts as a vertical gateway for the *shen* as they move between the Heavens and the Heart. As the *shen* settle, emotions are harmonized, a person centers in their own authentic being and the scattering effects of shock, trauma and excessive emotions are mitigated. Spirit Gate - *Shen Men* also opens horizontally from the Heart to the outer world. For this reason, it is a point of choice when there are issues related to interpersonal communication, relationship, intimacy and love. It is one of the main points I turn to when I want to activate the Heart's "feeling function," its innate intelligence and sense of appropriateness in the arena of relationship.

While all of the three Heart's ministers—the Small Intestine, Pericardium and Triple Heater—are involved in the formation of healthy boundaries and the protection of the Heart, the *shen* has its own innate tendency, which is to shine the light of the self out into the world without restriction or restraint. This innate tendency to shine, which we see so vividly expressed by a healthy child, is naturally modified over time by the Heart's capacity for discriminating wisdom or what the ancient Chinese spoke of as the Heart's rectitude and propriety—being appropriate in the deepest sense of knowing how to be and how to respond at any given time.[25]

The capacity to recognize the difference between danger and safety, the ability to create boundaries in relationships and a sense of right timing and behavior are hallmarks of a healthy Heart Monarch and are important spirit-level gifts of Spirit Gate - *Shen Men*.

I turn to this point to help a person discern whether or not it is safe to open the Heart's gate, when and how it is appropriate to shine the light of their spirit out into the world. It is also the point I turn to when this discernment has been damaged due to trauma or abuse or when the light has been dimmed by abandonment, betrayal or loss. Then the gentle healing wisdom of Spirit Gate - *Shen Men* can help to clear away the damaging residue of traumatic relationship experiences and open the way again for faith and trust when the conditions are favorable, and the boundaries are safe.

I turn to this point when I want to:

- call the scattered *shen* back to the nest of the Heart after shock, betrayal, loss, excess emotions and trauma

- balance mind and emotions; restore the meaningful connection between self and outer world

- balance the relationship between control and spontaneity

- calm hyper-vigilance, anxiety and agitation

- create a conduit of communication between the Heart and the mind

- enhance capacity for rest and receptivity; support restful sleep and dreams.

Suggested Essential Oil: Rose

Rose is the most important essential oil for the Heart and the Fire Element as a whole. There are at least 350 known rose species and over 10,000 hybrid varieties, but it is the single species, *Rosa damascene* or damask rose, cultivated since the 16th century, that is most prized for medicinal essential oil. It takes up to 60,000 roses to produce one small bottle of oil.

For over 5000 years, the rose has been a symbol of "love, in all its earthly and heavenly hues, what or who we love in the present, the one we have loved and have lost, and the longing for something nameless—embodied in the form and color of roses."[26] And yet the sweet fragrance and Divine beauty of the rose combines with a fierce thorniness that protects its exquisite and delicate blossom with sharp prickles. The potent combination of spiritual openness, alluring sweetness and beauty with assertive protectiveness and wise reticence is transmitted from the flower to the oil and becomes a balm for the many various wounds, scars and healings of the Heart.

When I use this oil, I feel that I am tapping into the wisdom of the plant in its fullest expression of discernment, caution, creativity, blossoming and trust. A drop of rose on Spirit Gate - *Shen Men* calls the scattered *shen* back to the Heart after shock, emotional upset and even excess states of joy, excitation and passion. The scent of the rose sends an ancient, archetypal message to the Heart that it is protected even when vulnerable, that there is strength in softness when combined with appropriate cunning and caution.

Rose oil is a cool, moist essence that provides gentle support and protection for the soul. It opens the Heart to love while at the same time augmenting the capacity for a critical assessment of safety and risk. It is particularly useful in the treatment of emotional wounds from loss, rejection and betrayal. It alleviates depression and restores a sense of wellbeing and joy. It allows me to be present to what is, rather than struggling to recover what is not.

The one caveat for rose oil is that it is crucial to find a good-quality, pharmaceutical-grade, unadulterated natural oil. Doing so can be quite expensive. However, a little bit goes a long way. A few drops dispersed in a carrier oil are, in most cases, sufficient for treatment and a small quarter-dram bottle can last up to a year if used judiciously.

Heart 8 - Lesser Mansion - *Shao Fu*
少府

This time of berries:
sweet sunlight kisses my tongue
with the taste of joy!

Opening the door to Heart 8 - Lesser Mansion - *Shao Fu* 少府 is like opening the door to the happiness of summer. Imagine lying against warm rocks in early August sun after a swim in cool water. Imagine gathering ripe blueberries in a basket, looking up and seeing a person you love also gathering nearby. No words are needed, just the sound of the breeze in the poplar leaves and the scent of berries in the sun.

Lesser Mansion - *Shao Fu* is about that kind of day, that kind of moment when the Heart is at peace, when the Fire is tended, when warmth and coolness, activity and rest, tranquility and joy, are in perfect equilibrium.

Lesser Mansion - *Shao Fu* is the *ying*-spring and Fire point of the Heart. It is commonly assumed that it is named for its location on the *shaoyin* or lesser yin channel. However, I feel that the character *shao* in the point name has other clues to tell us about the point's medicine. *Shao* 少 is a stylized picture of something small *xiao* 小 being further divided 丿 into something even smaller. It is used to mean small, few, tiny but also young, emergent. Taking this further, it points to something rare, precious and vulnerable.

Fu 府 means official residence or mansion. It is a picture of *guang* 广 a building or roof covering *fu* 付 a hand 寸 giving money or some other precious treasure to 亻a person. The radical *fu* 付 means pay, hand over or commit.

Lesser Mansion - *Shao Fu*, like all the *ying*-spring points, is recognized for its ability to clear heat. It's indicated specifically in cases where there are excess Heart Fire and heat, particularly for Heart heat that has traveled into the Small Intestine and Bladder meridians, resulting in mental restlessness, insomnia, emotional upset and dark, scanty and difficult urination. In addition, the point helps to regulate the qi of the Heart, whether deficient or stagnant. The dysregulation of Heart qi may be due to shock, acute or chronic relationship stress, mental exhaustion and constitutional weakness compounded with early childhood distress and trauma. Whatever the cause, the dysregulation of the Heart qi results in a wide variety of psycho-emotional disturbances, including anxiety, hysteria, labile emotions, palpitations and chest tightness.[27]

A closer look at the characters in the point name gives me a deeper insight into the spirit-level meaning of Lesser Mansion - *Shao Fu*. It tells me that this Fire within Fire point is a special "official" residence, where I can go to meet and directly communicate with the Monarch of the Heart. It also speaks of the point's capacity to support the Heart Monarch in handing over or spreading the rare and precious treasure of her radiance in an appropriately modulated way, without impediment or constriction, throughout the body, mind and spirit.

When I touch this point, I am touching the last stopping place before the spiritual influxes of the Heart disperse through Heart 9 - Little Rushing - *Shao Chong*, the exit point on the tip of the smallest finger. Whether I approach the point with a needle, oil, flower essence or expanded sight, I imagine I am opening the door to a small summer palace where the Empress of the Heart waits to meet me on her crimson throne. The Empress is easily startled and will scatter and hide if my approach is too loud or if I enter without invitation. But if I approach her with care and reverence, she comes forward to meet and receive me.

When the meeting is timely and the necessary rituals of approach are performed, the Monarch of the Heart, like summer sunlight, will naturally open her palm to hand over her precious treasures of warmth, joy, love, contentment and modulated passion. The peaceful look I see on my patient's face when the door to the palace is opened appropriately is enough to tell me of her blessing.

Suggested Flower Essence: Sandalwood

A drop of sandalwood at the door of Lesser Mansion - *Shao Fu* cools excess Fire and calms hyper-excitation of the Heart. It quiets over-active thoughts and helps to balance and harmonize the relationship between the Heart and the mind. It brings a quality of sacred stillness to the Palace that allows the Monarch to receive the celestial light that showers down on her in the form of insights and intuitions from Heaven.

Sandalwood oil has been recognized since antiquity as a rare, precious and sacred substance, a balm for the spirit and the soul. In the words of Gabriel Mojay, sandalwood "quells the mind as an incessant tool of analysis and expectation and...

frees it as a creative source, always present in the here and now. It is perhaps for this reason that it has been associated, in terms of the symbolism of the Tarot, with the Empress."[28]

Small Intestine 7 - Upright Branch - *Zhi Zheng*
支正

Resilient the green
leaves in a sea breeze dance
on the poplar's gnarled branches.

No sooner do the fire-orange blossoms irrupt from the green foliage of the Mexican sunflowers than the fritillary butterflies arrive. Seemingly out of nowhere, the creatures descend upon the flowers, their wings shivering with delight in the mid-summer breeze. They pause momentarily to gain purchase on the petals, then dip their delicate proboscces deep into the heart of the blossoms to siphon the pure, sweet nectar up into their nearly weightless bodies.

Attuned to the slightest vibration, they flutter and lift off into the sky if I approach too quickly. But moving slowly and stealthily, I can get close enough to see the intricate checker patterns for which they are named, the rhythmic alternation of black, orange, gold and fawn brown squares on their wings.

Now, I see their ephemeral fiery spirit, the *shen* that ignites them. I am delighted by their animation, light and beauty as they flutter their wings in the sun. But I also know that, deep within their epigenetic memory, there is another desire, another impulse, another Fire that arises from Tao, from the deepest origins of their being.

Within these sun-loving creatures of summer, there is an absolute knowing, a desire, direction and purpose that will guide them, at exactly the right moment, away from the sunlight in search of shade. In the cool, quiet corners of the garden, they will find the shy and tender violets where they will lay their thousands of tiny, translucent golden eggs. The larvae will sleep through the winter to awaken in spring at exactly the same time that the violets begin to grow. There the hungry caterpillars will feed on tender violet leaves. And there they will weave their cocoons and emerge as butterflies as the fire-orange blossoms with their sweet nectar irrupt once again, right on time, from the green foliage.

This unerring sense of rightness and timing, this knowing absolutely how to be and how to respond, this mysterious capacity to arrive at the right place at the right time... this is the virtue of the Heart, or what Taoists referred to as propriety—the Monarch's sense of absolute and appropriate alignment with Tao—expressed through the Small Intestine's virtue of discernment. This is the Heart's uprightness delivered by the hand of her minister, the Small Intestine. This is the excitation of Fire—desire, passion, radiance and beauty—extended through the generations as enduring illumination and the indomitable drive to create and procreate, express my own Divine purpose and manifest my Tao.

Small Intestine 7 - Upright Branch - *Zhi Zheng* 支正 is the *luo* junction point on the Small Intestine meridian. As *luo*, this point is where the channel spreads to connect with the Heart channel. It functions as the mediator between the yin and yang, interior and exterior aspects of the Fire Element. And it is the point where the Heart's inner radiance is mediated and extended out to the world by the Small Intestine.

The point name is composed of two characters. *Zhi* 支 is a stylized picture of *you* 又 a hand holding *shi* 十 a branch. *Zhi* is translated to mean branch, support, dispatch. It is also the word used in Chinese medicine to refer to the branching of a meridian. *Zheng* is derived from the word *zhi* 止 a picture of a left footprint, which means to stop. *Zheng* 正 is a picture of a foot with a line at the top indicating a step that arrives at the right place and stops at the right limit. It means correct, upright, exact and also to govern and rectify or make right.

On a physical level, Upright Branch - *Zhi Zheng* is indicated for inhibitions in arm, elbow, hand and finger mobility. It is also recognized for its ability to regulate and modulate communication between exterior and interior and to clear exterior heat pathogenic factors.[29] On a psycho-emotional level, it is indicated for the rectification of hyper-excitation and dysregulation of the Fire Element and the Heart, including symptoms such as anxiety, mania-depression, scattered mind, hysteria and restlessness.

Weaving together the various threads, we begin to understand the complex spirit-level power of the Upright Branch - *Zhi Zheng*. It supports the Small Intestine in standing guard at the Monarch's chamber and acting as protector of the Heart. However, the point also activates and regulates the Small Intestine's function as interpreter and communicator of the Monarch's messages. I consider this point when there is a need to rectify a person's behavior and communication. I call on it when the expression of emotion gets garbled or lost in translation or when communication takes the form of innuendo and inappropriate joking rather than clear, skillful transmission, particularly in the arena of sexuality, intimacy and love.

Many years ago, my first teacher, J. R. Worsley, mentioned the use of this point when there are sexual difficulties, including erectile dysfunction and declining libido. Reaching deeper, I recognize that the uprightness of this point lies in its yang capacity to serve as a righteous and steadfast conduit of communication between the yin Heart and the outer world. The point's spirit gift is found in its ability to support the Small Intestine in dispatching and appropriately disseminating the Heart's illuminating Fire and in helping me to recognize *kairos*—the right and opportune moment; the where, how and when to step; the extension of my *shen* into being, time and destiny.

Small Intestine 19 - Listening Palace - *Ting Gong*
聽宮

Crickets in the crimson
runner beans scratch ragged wings
against the moon.

Over dinner one summer evening, I asked some friends who run a small documentary theatre company to describe what listening means to them. They all agreed that distinguishing between hearing—an involuntary, neurological response to sound waves—and listening is primary.

For them, listening is a full-body experience that involves all the senses. It is a resonance that constellates between people. An exchange of energy. A hum in the air. Something comes to life that wasn't there before.

As activists dedicated to healing the wounds of community fragmentation and social divisiveness through talking to people from all walks of life around the country, my friends had discovered that listening doesn't just happen. It is a conscious practice. It is a skill that must be developed, cultivated and honed.

As I reflected on their words, I was struck by how relevant their experiences as artists and performers are to my own experiences in the treatment room. How many times has a patient told me, even before the insertion of a needle, that qi moved simply from my attentive listening? How many times has the treatment process shifted when I notice the grief beneath the laugh or the rage beneath the resigned sigh?

To listen beyond the words, to follow the arc of the emotion all the way to a person's soul—this is what allows us to recognize the poem, the dream, the riddle, the secret embedded in the case history. This listening is what allows us to move beyond the limits of the physical body and enter the sacred space of spirit-level healing.

In traditional Chinese medicine, the distinction between hearing and listening comes under the jurisdiction of the Small Intestine Official, the Separator of Pure from Impure, the Heart's closest minister. The Small Intestine's job is to sort through the barrage of information that comes at us from the outer environment and to recognize what is of true relevance to our own Heart. If we imagine the Heart as a Monarch seated on a throne at the center of our being, the Small Intestine is like the private secretary who appraises every piece of correspondence to determine if it is worthy of the Heart's attention. In order to fulfill this function, the Small Intestine must be able to sift through the infinite cacophony of impressions to discern the purest essences, the things that will bring us closer to our authentic nature—our Tao. In other words, the Small Intestine's job is to listen.

The central seat of this minister rests just in front of the ear and its name is Small Intestine 19 - Listening Palace - *Ting Gong* 聽宮. On the right side of the ancient character *ting* 聽 listening is the character *de* 德 virtue. This affirms for us the spiritual significance that the ancient Chinese ascribed to the act of listening. The presence of the radical *de* tells us that listening is a virtue, a defining quality of a truly engaged human, a hallmark of a sage.

And tucked away at the bottom of the character *de* is the radical *xin* 心 the Heart. The character tells us that when we touch this point, we are inviting a person to listen to the world as if the Heart is at the center.

Consider this point:

- when a person is unable to distinguish between the gold and the dross in their life

- when a person is overloaded with information and unable to make sense of it

- when the Fire Element's capacity to connect, communicate and relate to another is impaired by emotional tone-deafness

- when a person has forgotten how to hear their own music

- when there is a need to engage the Small Intestine's capacity for true empathy, to get as close as you possibly can to another person while always remembering that you are not them.

At this moment, wherever you are as you read these words, stop and place the tips of your fingers in the slight depression just in front of your ears and listen to the sounds around you.

Out of this tapestry of sound, find one sound: a voice outside the window, a footfall on a stair, a honking horn, sunlight on the sidewalk, a bird on a branch, a cloud passing, a star falling in a galaxy far, far away... Offer this sound as a gift to your Heart. Notice how your thoughts clear as you open this point, how something shifts as hearing becomes listening, how you enter a different kind of presence, how for a moment you recall the sacredness of the world around you.

You have just opened the door to the Heart. You have touched the spirit of the point of the Listening Palace - *Ting Gong*.

Suggested Flower Essence: Yarrow

The location of Listening Palace - *Ting Gong* at the sensitive skin in front of the tragus of the ear makes it a good choice for flower essence application. I think of yarrow flower essence in connection with Listening Palace - *Ting Gong*, as both essence and point have to do with discriminating listening—the ability to sift through incoming impressions and separate the grain from the chaff.

Master flower essence practitioners and teachers Patricia Kaminski and Richard Katz write that yarrow flower essence "literally knits together the overly porous aura...so that it does not 'bleed' excessively into the environment...and bestows a shining shield of Light which protects and unifies the essential Self..."[30] I call on yarrow to support and strengthen the Small Intestine's ability to discriminate between impressions that are energetically life-affirming and nourishing to the Heart and input that is toxic. A drop of this flower essence at the door of the Listening Palace - *Ting Gong* reminds the Small Intestine minister of the crucial importance of his tasks: separating pure from impure, protecting the Monarch from distracting, depleting data and creating a shield between devitalizing influences from the environment and the vibrant radiance of the *shen*.

Pericardium 8 - Palace of Weariness - *Lao Gong*
勞宮

Now, only the touch
of a green dragonfly wing
ripples this peaceful pond.

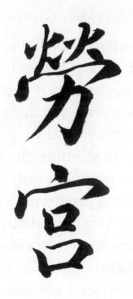

At the high point of Summer, a crimson poppy bursts from its green bud and brings to fullness the promise of its minute black seed. This moment of flowering, this fleeting time of peak summer, arrives with a surprising clamor of color and then, almost before we catch a glimpse of its beauty, begins to soften and fade under the downward pull of the yin. The petals of the poppy fall and the ovule of the flower grows heavy, swelling to form the pod and seeds that will become its harvest.

The profusion of summer's blooming and the exuberant yang thrusting of the life force upward toward the light reminds me of my own desire to flourish, to be recognized and admired as I take the risk of blossoming the seed of my innermost nature out into the world. But the transience of summer also reminds me of my vulnerability, my susceptibility to the effects of time and atmosphere and my dependence on the nourishing potency of the yin—the rejuvenating power of rest and rootedness—in order for the radiance of my spirits to shine in a stable and ongoing way. Like the poppy, I need the yang invitation of sunlight to incite my blossoming, but also the yin wrapping of the bud to protect me as I grow.

Pericardium 8 - Palace of Weariness - *Lao Gong* 勞宮 is the Fire in the Fire point on the Pericardium meridian. It is a point that expresses Fire's paradox—its capacity to reach outward, to blossom, expand, connect, activate and illuminate and its vulnerability, its need to curl inward for protection, cultivation and care. The point is considered a central vortex of energy in *qi gong* and is recognized in Chinese medicine as having profound emotional and spiritual effects. It functions as a doorway that can open but also close, a point that can invigorate but also sedate. It is a safe house, a nest where the Heart spirit can go for rest and restoration.

The point name is made up of the character *lao* 勞 meaning labor, toil or weariness and the character *gong* 宮 which translates as palace, but is also used to refer to the womb or uterus.[31] *Lao* 勞 combines 熒, a picture of two flames over a roof, above the radical *li* 力 strength. *Gong* 宀 is a picture of a roof over 呂 a window and a door. Taken together, the two characters reinforce the importance of a protective covering for the wellbeing of the Fire Element. Without protection, the flame of the Heart is easily destabilized and even extinguished. Our inner strength is lost and the creative, protective and life-engendering Fires of the womb are threatened. For me, the fact that the graphic for *lao* 勞 is made up of two flames rather than just one affirms the idea that the Heart's strength arises from relationship—either to oneself or another—and that the creation and maintenance of appropriate relational boundaries (the roof, window and door) are key to caring for our Fire.

The great seventh-century Taoist scholar and physician Sun Simiao includes Palace of Weariness - *Lao Gong* on the list of the Thirteen Ghost Points[32] in his *Thousand Ducat Formula*.[33] The physician recognized the special ability of these 13 points to effectively treat psycho-emotional issues. He believed that without adequate protection, the Heart and *shen* are susceptible to invasion by excess emotion and worries and also toxic psychic energies. These invasive pathogenic factors transform into a kind of phlegm possession that clouds our capacity to see who we really are or what we are meant to accomplish. The Ghost Points clear away the mists of phlegm and the *gui* who hang about in the dampness. In addition, these points also offer protection and illumination so that the spirit can shine once again.

In its function as a Ghost Point, Palace of Weariness - *Lao Gong* is known by its alternative name, *Gui Ku* 鬼窟 Ghost Cave. When I call on it for its Ghost Point wisdom, I am looking to help a person retrieve their own resources that are hidden in the cave of unconsciousness. I want to help them clear away the fog of misconception and fear so that they can see their own light and feel their own authentic passion.

Of all the points in the body, this is the one that I find most supports the paradoxical human desire to open to self and others and, at the same time, maintain a safe boundary between the Heart and the outer world. In this regard, its placement on the cross point of the hand, the "crucifixion point" at the center of the palm, seems particularly significant. The point's location symbolically confirms its capacity to help us bear the tension of opposites that is so much a part of the experience of embodiment and to live more consciously on the cross of matter.

Another aspect of this point's wisdom is simply its capacity to activate a protective, semi-permeable membrane, a shield around the Heart that allows positive energies and love to enter the Monarch's chamber while effortlessly deflecting toxic or negative influences. I often give my patients an essential oil or flower essence to apply to this point themselves when they're going through a challenging relationship process or before and after a highly charged meeting or interpersonal exchange.

I open the door to the Palace of Weariness - *Lao Gong* when I want to offer a patient a safe haven to heal from trauma or loss. As I needle the point, I imagine that I am bringing them to a place of seclusion and safety, where, after a time of convalescence, they can gather strength and come back to their own center.

This point offers a feeling of protection, particularly when a person has shared deeply during a session. After an intense emotional experience or significant opening in the treatment room, the Palace of Weariness - *Lao Gong* provides a sense of strength and appropriate shielding without rigid shutdown. A few cones of moxa or a drop of essential oil on this point help my patients to integrate and process the energetic shifts of an intense treatment in a more manageable way.

I see the Palace of Weariness - *Lao Gong* as a translucent dome of ruby-colored glass through which the diffused sunlight shines down to warm and calm the *shen*, a refuge when the outer world becomes too much for the spirit to bear. It is not a place to hide or to deny the exigencies of life, but rather a sacred place of prayer, a protected space where we can return to our own black seed and rediscover the Divine spark of our spirit's Heavenly mandate. In the hushed silence and peace that comes after the point is touched, space opens where the Heart can rest.

Suggested Treatment Strategy: Less is More!

This is a potent and highly responsive point. Due to its location on the acutely sensitive palm of the hand, I have found that less stimulation is very often more. I needle it with a fine-gauge needle when deeper stimulation is required. Otherwise, I turn to gentler tools. A single rice grain moxa burned directly on the point is sometimes sufficient to make the necessary shift. I rarely use more than three grains.

The point responds beautifully to: rose essential oil which calms the *shen* and provides protection and healing for the Heart; blue tansy for clearing, releasing intrusive energies and strong spirit protection; lavender to brighten and uplift the soul.

Pericardium 9 - Rushing into the Middle - *Zhong Chong*

中衝

What beauty! The blue
returning tide, swirling over
these hot summer stones.

Pericardium 9 - Rushing into the Middle - *Zhong Chong* 中衝 arrives with a surprise, like the first day when spring turns to summer, the day you rush outside to feel the sudden joy, the brightness of the light, the freedom of bare feet in the grass and warm air against your skin.

As the Wood in the Fire point on the Pericardium meridian, Rushing into the Middle - *Zhong Chong* is about adding fuel to the Fire. It activates the qi, circulates the blood and enlivens the *shen*.

Zhong 中 is a picture of a square with a vertical line through its center. It is often described as an arrow flying straight to the heart of a target. The energy of the graphic captures the flawless accuracy of the aim, the division of the single square into two equal parts. Even the sound of the pronunciation—*chonnnng*—communicates a feeling of activation, vibration, vitality, direction and fast change. *Zhong* is translated to mean middle, center, interior, the passing of an exam or succeeding at a task; something that strikes and perfectly pierces a target.

Chong 衝 combines the radical *xing* 行 a picture of two footprints, also described as a crossroad, with the phonetic *zhong* 重 a picture of a pile of flat weights. *Xing* 行 means to move forward and through. It means, "Okay! Let's go!" *Zhong* 重 means to rush toward something, to vigorously charge, dash, clash, collide, to put all my weight behind my action and give it the power of my full force.

The energy of Rushing into the Middle - *Zhong Chong* is definitive, clear, swift and direct. When I needle this point, I am calling on the Pericardium Official to bring forth the full, directed force of her power as protector, circulator, minister, master and manifester of the Monarch of the Heart.

We say that the Heart is essentially void because the void gives it the potential to receive the directives and illumination of the *shen* and to become the dwelling place of the spirit. But in order for the invisible emanations of the void of the Heart spirit to have an actual effect, there must be a way for the radiance to have embodied expression. This active aspect of the Heart's charge of sovereignty is carried out by the Pericardium, "that other aspect of the heart, that which manifests its power on the middle finger, the longest and largest finger...the one who is in charge of accomplishing things...whether governing a country or organizing a banquet."[34]

Rushing into the Middle - *Zhong Chong*, like all *jing*-well points, clears heat and restores consciousness. It is also recognized for its connection to self-expression, its ability to "loosen the tongue," to allow me to speak the truth of my Heart and to communicate my deepest feelings with clarity to those I am intimate with.

As the primary tonification point of *xin bao luo*—the Pericardium in her role as Heart Protector—this point brings warmth and viability to the vessel matrix, the envelope of qi and blood, the womb-like wrapper that energetically surrounds and protects the Heart and *shen*. As the vitalizer of *tan zhong*—the Pericardium in her role as master of the center—the point moves qi through the chest and circulates the blood so that it can travel freely from the Heart out through the arteries to the limbs' smallest micro-vessels. Through the protection of the Heart and the liberated flow of qi and blood, I am empowered to manifest the warmth, spirit and joy and the appropriate actions, speech and self-governance that are the radiance of Heaven within me.

Suggested Treatment Strategy: Rice Grain Moxa

Rushing into the Middle - *Zhong Chong*, like all nail points, can be painful and a bit shocking to the Heart. If activated carelessly or with undue force, we risk scattered *shen* and a traumatized patient! I always give people a little warning before needling this point and use the smallest needle to get the job done. When the Fire is overheated, resulting in signs such as heatstroke, agitation and restlessness, strong needling is necessary and, in rare cases, it may even be useful to carefully bleed the nail point. When excess Fire clears through this point, the relief feels like the returning blue tide pouring over hot summer stones.

When the Fire is low, resulting in sadness, oppression, instability of mood, deficient circulation of warmth and lack of joy, I find that a slower, gradual activation of the point is more effective. In cases of deficiency or stasis, the application of three to five direct rice grain moxa, pausing in between to allow the Heart to absorb the heat as it passes back to the chest through the Pericardium, tonifies and stabilizes the Fire. Watch for color and pulse changes and be careful not to overtreat. Remember, this point responds with a rush and less is often more. If three moxa get at it, stop there! You may not even need to needle to get the desired effect.

Triple Heater 5 - Outer Frontier Gate - *Wai Guan*
外關

Fling open the gate.
Here comes the wind. This evening's
welcome visitor.

From early dawn to last late light, the cacophony continues in the form of bird song, cicada whirr, mosquito buzz until it turns dark and becomes a hum: the flickering code communication of fireflies, the snuffling and stamping of deer and thrumming of tree frogs. Torrents of smelts chased by seals, diving kingfishers and gulls, eagles harassing ospreys in the cove. And in the garden, cucumber vines curling and tumbling over carrots and mustard greens, roses seducing honeybees with fragrance and the photo-sensitive network of leaves, twigs and branches intertwining in their search for the sun.

Summer. It's all about connection and communication. I open the door and step outside, allowing myself to fully experience the complexity of impressions that infiltrate my senses: the threads of sound, scent, sensation and color that weave together the fabric of connection between the world and me.

Sometimes it's too much! It's all I can do to just be present, to walk out into the evening and watch the Thunder Moon rise over the pine trees.

Triple Heater 5 - Outer Frontier Gate - *Wai Guan* 外關, the *luo*-connecting point on the Triple Heater meridian, is a point for this kind of high summer day when the Fire Element is at its peak. It is a point that manages the entry and exit of information into and out of my being, that helps to harmonize and regulate the flow of impressions and maintain the appropriate heat and intensity of relationships. Outer Frontier Gate - *Wai Guan* epitomizes the virtue of the Triple Heater Official, the aspect of Fire that has to do with appropriate communication amongst and between, within and without. The point supports the Triple Heater's function as gatekeeper, the official in charge of the drawbridge that links the palace of my inner kingdom to the world.

Wai 外 contains the radical *xi* 夕, a picture of a crescent moon, which means evening, and *bu* 卜, a crack on the outside of a tortoiseshell, which means fortune-telling or divination. Together, the two radicals imply a ritual that happens under the moon, outside the limits of daylight and ordinary time. *Wai* is translated to mean outside or exterior but also foreign and excluded.

Guan 關 is a picture of 門 two leaves of a door or gate

combined with 絲 the silk threads radical. The graphic implication of the character is of two doors sealed by a woven matrix of threads. It implies a barrier that is sturdy but not impervious. The character is used to mean shut, locked, crux, passageway or turning point, but also a customs house or frontier pass at the outer edges of a kingdom.

When I choose to open the Outer Frontier Gate - *Wai Guan*, I call up the image of an ancient Chinese palace, connected to the countryside by a drawbridge that crosses a moat and opens to a weaving of waterways, rivers, streams, ditches and irrigation channels. All communications and all deliveries of goods and services are carried by boats of all sizes—rowboats, sampans, coracles, junks and merchant vessels—that travel back and forth through the connecting threads of Water. The Triple Heater Official is "responsible for the opening up of these passages and irrigation."[35] The *luo* point of this meridian, Outer Frontier Gate - *Wai Guan*, further refines this opening of passages and regulates the flow between the outer yang world of the Triple Heater and the inner yin world of the Pericardium.

Conventionally, this point is indicated for symptoms having to do with temperature regulation and the management of flow between interior and exterior on physical and sensory levels. It is used to release the exterior, benefit the head and ears, clear heat and activate the channel. Typical symptoms include chills due to injury by cold, headache, impaired hearing, eye swelling and redness, difficulty speaking, constipation, arm pain and stiffness, including the inability to grasp objects.[36]

On a spirit level, I consider this point when a person is having difficulty maintaining even flow between their inner world and the environment. This can take the form of cut-off loneliness, as with a person terrified by public speaking or too shy to promote their own work, who is unable to receive the nourishment they need from relationships, unable to take hold of and make good use of the objects of the outer world. But it can also take the form of hyperactive communication, such as a fiery extroverted political person who is completely exhausted by too many speeches, too many cocktail parties, too many handshakes. In both cases, the official in charge of the Outer Frontier Pass is having difficulty managing the flow. Calling on the wisdom and medicine of Outer Frontier Gate - *Wai Guan* can help clear the waterways and regulate communication between within and without.

As the *luo* point, Outer Frontier Gate - *Wai Guan* also connects the extroverted and introverted aspects of the Fire Element, the yang Triple Heater with the yin Pericardium. In this way, it has a tempering effect on the emotions and moderate intake of sensory impressions, so that the cacophony of over-yang, over-active communication is harmonized and modulated by the softer, lunar wisdom of the moon. Then, my Heart can listen rather than simply hear what the world is telling me. I can "divine" the meaning of the signs and take in the music of the spirit that sings to me from the natural world.

Suggested Essential Oil: Vetiver

Vetiver essential oil is made from grasses that flourish on the slopes of the Himalayan mountains in southern India and Malaysia. The thickly entangled mats of the fragrant, spongy rootlets of the plant are dug up, washed, dried and distilled to produce the oil. The fibrous roots have also been used for centuries to thatch roofs and in the weaving of curtains on doors as well as for the blinds and screens of Indian households. The roots darken the blinds and shield the interior of the houses from the sun. In the heat of high summer, the curtains, blinds and screens are doused with water. As they dry, they add fragrance to the breezes that pass through the blinds. This fragrant breeze not only cools the interior of the house but also repels bugs.

The yin, cooling, moistening and protective qualities that the rootlets bring to Indian households are also present in the essential oil. Vetiver has a regulating effect as it sedates and strengthens the nervous system. It can be used to calm a hyperactive mind and help restore and replenish a spirit that is overwhelmed and exhausted by yang outer activity. It heals the damage done to the nerves by shock, fear and stress, harmonizes dysregulated emotions and alleviates insomnia and dream-disturbed sleep. It is also known to enhance and regulate the libido and the flow of sexual energies and can be useful in helping to heal frigidity and sexual anxiety.

When there is hypervigilance, a drop of vetiver on the Outer Frontier Gate - *Wai Guan* can be called on to reduce the outward-directed defensive action. And when there is excess porousness, the oil supports the Triple Heater in creating a gentle yet effective screen between the Heart and the outer world.

Conception Vessel 15 - Dove Tail - *Jiu Wei*

尾鳩

In the tender light
of this early-summer dawn,
my heart door opens.

My first experience of this point was shortly after the death of my father. I was overcome by grief as if the world was covered in a mist of sadness. Just a few weeks earlier, I had told him of my decision to apply to acupuncture school and he had given me his blessing. So it was with a heavy Heart that I realized he would not be there to see me complete my training and begin what was to become my lifelong work.

When my acupuncturist inserted the needle into the point, I was surprised to feel a clearing open in the mists of my tears. My diaphragm released and my breathing deepened. A tingling light streamed through my chest and abdomen. The gray clouds within me became tinged with rose and gold. I remembered the feeling of being a child at my father's side, listening to the stories of the Monkey King and Princess Aurora Borealis that he made up especially for me. Two divergent rivers of emotion—grief from my Lungs and grateful joy from my Heart—had joined into a single, beautiful braided flow of healing.

On a physical level, Conception Vessel 15 - Dove Tail - *Jiu Wei* 尾鳩 is located at the tip of the xiphoid process, the meeting point where the two sides of the rib cage come together. The sternum is said to be the back of the dove, the ribs her wings and the xiphoid her tail.

Its location lies midway between the umbilicus, where the prenatal energies of *wu shen* enter the fetus, and the Heart, where the *shen* is ultimately installed as the organizer and guide of our postnatal existence. This in-between area is referred to in ancient medical texts as the *gao* 膏 and Dove Tail - *Jiu Wei* is mentioned in the *Spiritual Pivot* as its source point.[37] For this reason, acupuncturist and scholar Dennis Willmont refers to Dove Tail - *Jiu Wei* as the "Spirit Transmitter," the arbiter between pre- and postnatal energies and the "final point of the inception of the *shen* into the physical body."[38] Willmont speaks of Dove Tail - *Jiu Wei* as the circulation point where the prenatal Kidney Waters of Destiny and the postnatal Heart Fires of Human Nature interpenetrate in an ongoing tidal ebb and flow. However, due to excess or held-back emotion, the smooth flow of the Kidney Water and Heart Fire through the *gao* may be impeded. Then, stuck fluids and knotted qi congeal into a fat, greasy substance also called *gao*.

Ancient physicians recognized the serious dangers of accumulated *gao*[39] in the subcostal region and emphasize the difficulty in treating disease once it has settled in this area.[40] Texts underscore the influence of stress, emotional constraint and excessive sexual activity in the etiology of this problem. However, ancient alchemists understood that *gao*, while toxic in its raw state, could transform into a potent medicinal paste or salve when it is worked with in the right way. This tells me that releasing the accumulated energies of the *gao* through lifestyle changes, inner work and timely and appropriate activation of Dove Tail - *Jiu Wei* can help to release knotted emotions that have accumulated in the chest, free up the life force and support a person in finding their way back to clarity and true life purpose.

Dove Tail - *Jiu Wei* is the front-*mu* 募 collecting point of the Pericardium, and it allows us to directly access, raise and gather the wisdom of the Heart Protector Official. When needled skillfully, the point supports the Pericardium's capacity to protect the Heart from pathogenic influences while allowing positive energies to nourish the *shen*. In addition, the point can help to calm the spirit, clear away phlegm obscuring the Heart, release congealed qi in the chest and distribute vitalizing qi, fluids and essences through the fascial sheaths and energetic pathways of the abdomen.

This is a point to consider when a person is caught at an emotional impasse, especially when struggling with the opposing impulses to both open and protect the Heart. When a person is recovering from loss or betrayal, this point will bring a sense of acceptance and release. When there are intimacy issues, relationship-related states of anxiety and worry along with feelings of overwhelm and hysteria, the point will bring a sense of trust and calm. Also consider this point when a person is struggling with timidity, avoidance of social contact, distrust of self and others and sexual difficulties related to fear of intimacy.

Suggested Essential Oil: Spikenard

Dove Tail - *Jiu Wei* welcomes direct rice grain moxa, gentle moxa pole heat and sensitive touch. I also find it very responsive to the application of essential oils and flower essences. One of my oils of choice for this point is Himalayan spikenard or Jatamansi. This is the oil said to have been used by Mary Magdalene in the anointing of Jesus's feet. Centuries earlier, it was used by early Egyptian priests, Hindu adepts and Ayurvedic doctors for ritual and pharmaceutical purposes.

Spikenard has a harmonizing effect on the nervous system and a calming effect on the *shen*. It supports relaxation, brings restful sleep and can help regulate Heart rhythm. For me, this oil's most important effects arise from its honey-sweet yet spicy aroma and its viscous consistency yet translucent amber color, which, like the alchemical *gao*, endow it with the paradoxical qualities of weight and buoyancy. I find that spikenard can both coagulate and root untethered yang Fire and liberate, lift, aerate and disperse collapsed yin Water. It offers a feeling of safety and protection while clearing phlegm and opening the orifices to connection with the world. In this way, it supports the free flow of both yin and yang and the movement of Tao.

I consider the application of spikenard to Dove Tail - *Jiu Wei* when a person is recovering from loss, emotional wounding, betrayal in a relationship and destabilizing life changes. When the *shen* has been dislodged from the palace of the heart, a drop of this ancient golden oil will guide the Monarch gently back to her rightful place on the throne at the center, protected by her ministers, rooted in the blood and illuminated by the stars.

Bladder 38 (or 43) - Rich for the Vitals - *Gao Huang Shu*

膏肓俞

My heart breaks open,
as a single osprey's cry
pierces the blue twilight.

For years, each August evening as I returned from my kayak trip out to Darling Island, I would put down my paddle and pause for a few moments at the edge of a small, rocky promontory at the head of the harbor. Summer after summer, as the sun would set and the clouds turned to rose, lavender and gold ribbons in the west, without fail a lone black silhouette would lift off from the peak of the highest pine, career above my head and fly out over the water.

Then, the call would come, the long piercing cry that ricocheted off the rocks, echoed over the waves and filled the bowl of the darkening sky to the brim. This was our sacred meeting, a kind of agreement between me and the natural world that, despite dire warnings about weather chaos, species extinction and ever-increasing doubts about the possibility of a "cure" for the planet's degrading environment, certain rituals would remain. I would paddle out to the small island each summer afternoon and on my return, the sea hawk would be waiting at the promontory to welcome me home before going out on her twilight hunt.

Then, one summer, she was gone. I paddled back at dusk and waited at the point, but no careening silhouette rose from the trees, no wild hunter's cry ricocheted from the rocks.

She's still not back. Each summer, my boat gets a bit heavier and my paddle more challenging. But I continue to go out, and on my return at twilight, I wait at the promontory and hope to catch a glimpse of her, hope to hear her sharp whistle rising in the wind. And even later, when my ashes blow out to sea with the ragged breezes, I will listen for her sound, the single cry at twilight that breaks my Heart and cracks open the evening stars.

Bladder 38 (or 43) - Rich for the Vitals - *Gao Huang Shu* 膏肓俞 is a point for this kind of heartbreak and loss, for ancient wounds, debilitating depletion, chronic coldness, agitation, despair, emotional isolation and deep-seated diseases. Located on the outer Bladder line parallel to Bladder 14, the Pericardium back-*shu* point, I consider this point to be a doorway to the spirit of the Pericardium. I also regard it as a partner point to the Conception Vessel 15 - Dove Tail - *Jiu Wei*, the Pericardium's front-*mu* point. These two points are known for their capacity to unbind the chest, calm the spirit and clear phlegm from the Heart. Even more remarkably, they are two of the few points known to move qi and blood through the microchannels of the *Gao Huang*, the "deepest and most fundamental region of the body"[41] located between the Heart and diaphragm where the fluids of unexpressed emotions congeal and chronic and incurable illnesses are said to lodge.[42]

As noted in the previous entry, *gao* is both the name of the tender inner pericardial tissues located immediately beneath the Heart and a kind of rich, viscous, fatty, creamy substance that has both pathogenic and healing properties. The character *gao* 膏 is a picture of *ting* 亭 a high tower or a presiding capital building above *rou* 月, meaning flesh. The character graphically describes the position of the *gao* at the high point of the breastbone just beneath the Monarch's palace and also its power of jurisdiction over the flesh and blood as well as other vital organs.

Huang 肓 combines *wang* 亡 (originally drawn as 凵), which is described as a picture of a person stuck in a corner or hiding place and means to lose or die, with the radical *rou* 月 flesh. *Huang* refers to the region of the vitals, the area of the body between the *gao* and the bottom of the diaphragm. The underlying graphic meaning of the character affirms the vital life-death significance of this area to the wellbeing of the body, mind and spirit. In fact, the word *gaohuang* can be used to mean something that is beyond cure.

Shu 俞 is a picture of *zhou* 舟 a little boat or ferry barge going along upstream on *shui* 巛 the water.

Combining the three characters of the point name, I understand that Rich for the Vitals - *Gao Huang Shu* is a transport point that moves qi and blood between the middle and lower aspects of the thorax. It is the alchemical mixing point that can transform pathologically stuck *gao* into life-giving qi, circulating blood and accessible emotions. It is the master point of the web matrix of the *xin bao luo*—the Pericardium in her role as protector of the Heart and uterine sheath of the embryo of the *shen* spirit. And it is the regulating point of the *tan zhong*—the Pericardium in her role as master of the center, resident and envoy of the Sea of Qi in the chest and circulator of the blood.

Located on the outer Bladder line on the back, this point is often overlooked in modern practice. And yet it is a point to consider for many of the conditions that plague our world:

insomnia, mania, asthma, low sexual energy, palpitations and undiagnosable chronic diseases. Going deeper, I would say that it is a point for the enfeebled soul of our time, the lack of intimacy and emotional warmth, blockages in the flow of feeling, debilitating isolation and loneliness and the sense that life itself has lost its coherence and meaning.

I hold this point close to my Heart as I wait for my friend the osprey's return and envision it healing our planet's seemingly incurable ills. After all, in the words of the revered ancient physician, Sun Simiao, "there is no disorder that this point cannot treat."[43]

Suggested Treatment Strategy: Moxa Cones

Rich for the Vitals - *Gao Huang Shu* is a point that responds to warmth and Fire! Classical texts recommend 100 and even as many as 300 cones. In the words Sun Simiao, "once moxibustion is completed, it causes a person's yang to be healthy and full."[44] Some texts forbid needle stimulation, but I find that the point responds well to judicious needling in combination with moxa.

While 300 moxa cones may be more than my own fingers can sustain at this point in my practice, I do not hold back when it comes to warming this point. What is important is that I stay in close relationship to my patient as I perform the treatment. It is not only the heat of the moxa but also the healing warmth of connection and relationship that will ultimately cure the incurable diseases of our time.

Earth: Late Summer Season

Earth season arrives, expected but still taking my body by surprise. Summer's Fire is dying down—not yet to embers but to a softer flame. I walk out into the cool, damp garden and I feel a humid heaviness come over me. The sunflowers can barely hold up their golden heads. The squash has swollen overnight to inedible sizes and I feel the weight of time settling on my shoulders. The ghosts of Autumn are still hidden behind the curtain of the green world but I hear their preparations, the rustling of their skirts and jackets as they stretch and yawn in their underworld beds and the snapping of twigs as they pick the dry dirt from underneath their fingernails.

The Chinese character for Earth is *tu* 土. The downward-directed, stabilizing, rootedness of Earth is graphically expressed by this picture, which is said to represent a clod of soil or a plant rooting deep into the ground.

The Earth Element comes in Late Summer, at the waning of the warm days, the time of harvest and gathering. Its placement is on the top right of the *sheng* cycle, the point where the qi tips over the top and down the other side. As we move from the left to the right side of the Wheel, the entropic pull of gravity increases as the upward lift of heat and light decrease. There is more moisture, more matter, more weight. The dynamic catalyzing energies of the yang are limited by the formative and fixing tendencies of the yin. Through this limiting of yang spirit by yin matter, the exuberant creativity of Fire coagulates, contracts and transforms into the generous, nourishing bounty of Earth.

Kigo words evoke the hazy, golden atmosphere of Late Summer, of ripening and gathering, harvest, abundance and repletion. Mist softens the edges of the meadow grass at dawn. Song sparrows peck for fallen coneflower seeds. Gourds split open and the scent of apples fills the air as bees buzz drowsily over hedges of spiky purple thistle. Sunlight spills over the lip of early afternoon like sweet peaches pouring from a basket. Earth season arrives on a slow and humid morning, calling us to nourish ourselves and each other, to celebrate the generosity of the land. Yet, as the season cycle tips back down to darkness, Earth reminds us that unless we enjoy and share her gifts, they will ultimately end up rotting in the field. Earth calls us to give and to receive, to assimilate, transform and deliver while we digest.

Vegetative Expression

Earth's vegetative expression is the fruit of the vine, the parts of plants and trees where the capacity to sustain and nourish life is produced and gathered. The fruit stabilizes and incarnates the yang vitality of the sunlight that has poured down on the plant through summer. It allows this fiery yang vitality to become available to other beings in the form of food. But unless the products of the Earth season are actively used, eaten, transformed and digested by another being, they will rot or desiccate and not be able to express the generous nature that is their Tao. Thus, in Earth's mantra, "I nourish," we already hear the faint whisper of Metal: "I surrender to transformation."

Color/Sound/Odor/Emotion

The Color of Earth is Yellow

In the *Neijing Suwen*, we read, "Yellow is the color of the center; it pervades the spleen and lays open the mouth and retains the essential substances with the spleen."[1] To diagnose the health of the Earth, look at the sides of the eyes, temples and laugh lines around the mouth for a range of yellow from ripe grain to daffodil to goldfinch wing. The text further tells us, "When their color is yellow like that of oranges they are without life... When their color is yellow like the belly of a crab they are full of life."[2]

The Sound is Sing

The singing sound has an up-and-down energetic that is an auditory expression of the harmonizing, balancing nature of this Element. The singing sound is one that naturally arises when we are called to nurture others and is often heard when a mother is speaking to her young child. In imbalance, the singing sound can veer toward a whine or repetitive sing-song. In health, it is a sound that brings an atmosphere of gracious calm and generous good nature.

The Odor is Fragrant

In balance, the fragrant odor is like the smell of honey, ripe apples or fresh flower petals. However, despite its appealing name, an out-of-balance fragrant is just as disturbing as any of the other odors. In a pathological state, fragrant can be as cloying and sickly sweet as gardenia flowers in a warm room, old leather shoes in a closed closet or excess perfume.

The Emotion is Sympathy

In health, sympathy is a thoughtful, empathic attitude toward self and others. We can get as close as possible to another person or to ourselves while maintaining a conscious boundary, a breathing space that allows a process to unfold. In imbalance, sympathy becomes enmeshment and fusion. The breathing space collapses and transformational processes stall and bog down in pathological entropy.

The Officials

The main function of the two Earth Officials is to allow us to digest our life experiences and to use them in service to Tao. They are "responsible for the storehouses and granaries,"[3] the gathering and the assimilation and distribution of nutrients at every level of our being.

The Stomach Official is called the Official of Rotting and Ripening of Food and Drink. It breaks down the physical food and the experiences and ideas that we take in so that the essences can be transformed into various states of qi. J. R. Worsley compares the Stomach's activity to a concrete mixer. However, he qualifies this statement to say that the action of the Stomach is not simply a passive grinding but rather requires the official's judicious assessment of how ingredients need to be mixed for the proper nourishment of the body, mind and spirit.[4] The understanding is that the Stomach is responsible for the macerating and correct processing of the ingredients—food and fluids and concepts, experiences and ideas—so that we have the correct mixture for our health, strength and wellbeing, and ultimately our ability to manifest our authentic nature and Tao.

The Spleen Official is the Official of Transportation and Distribution. This Official's task is to direct the transportation of the qi that is derived from the essences to where it is needed. It is like a traffic director who stands at the center of a crossroads and guides the deliveries of goods to the appropriate parts of the body, mind and spirit. On a psycho-spiritual level, the Spleen's task is to process the experiences and information we receive and, through its capacity for critical distinction and reflection, transform the raw material of experience into potent ideas and activated imagination. At the center of all movement, the Spleen Official stands in calm repose at the neutral point—the spiritual pivot—where the possibilities of Heaven become manifest as realities on Earth.

Yi: The Spirit of Earth

The spirit of the Earth Element is the *yi* 意, translated as intention. The *yi* represents the quality of determined and clear intention and purpose that is at the core of a healthy Earth Element. During our lives, this spirit resides in the Spleen and is the animating force of our physical, emotional and spiritual muscle—our capacity to transform our potential visions, plans and intentions into empowered action and form in the material world. The *yi* is related to the Third or Solar Plexus Chakra and our potency, our power, our ability to burn the fuel of food and life energy so that we can "do" what we need to do. It is also related to the Fifth or Throat Chakra, our capacity to receive nurturance and to speak the words of our Hearts out to the world, to declare our truth and then to do it. The *yi*, like the Third and Fifth Chakras, supports our ability to "walk our talk" and to manifest our true destiny.

The *yi* is the aspect of our psyches that allows us to think clearly, study and appropriately digest and retain the information that we receive. It is also the spirit in charge of ideas, the concentration of the mind and the mental capacity to analyze—to break down and make use of information.

Beyond all that, it is the intention in us that allows us to manifest potential. Its presence is so all-encompassing that it is easy to overlook the spirit of the Earth, to neglect to honor its needs and the vital processes it regulates. The *yi* is not a potent mysterious force like the *zhi*, a winged visionary like the *hun* or a resplendent monarch like the *shen*. Rather, it's like a humble craftsperson or a devoted gardener who stays with the work—the planting, hoeing, weeding and watering—until the seeds of the garden have sprouted, grown and blossomed, and the harvest is ready to be enjoyed.

The character for *yi* 意 intent is made up of two parts: *xin* 心, the open bowl of the Heart placed below the radical *yin* 音, indicating an uttered sound, poetry or a musical note. From the etymology, we see that *yi* gives us the power not only to sing the music of our Hearts but also to continue to apply ourselves to our singing until our words and actions have crystallized into form.

In the sacred mountain that is the symbol of the self, the *yi* resides in the fertile fields at the horizon line between the upper mountain and the underworld. Unlike the other four spirits, the *yi* does not have an allegiance to Above or Below. Rather, it is the balance point, the place where opposites meet in service of transformation. The *yi* holds the position of the central axis between idea and action. It is the spirit in charge of the middle ground where the Tao of my life unfolds.

Earth's spirit question: Are my words and my actions in integrity with each other?

Spirit Animal: The Phoenix

The spirit of the Spleen has the form of the Phoenix. The Phoenix's given name is Hall of the *Hun* Soul and its spirit name is Constant Presence. Its given name tells us something about the role of the *yi* spirit in giving containment and concrete substance to the visions of the *hun*. For the *hun*'s abstract plans to begin to come into concrete form, the persevering tenacity and potent muscularity of the *yi* is necessary. The essential quality that gives rise to the Earth's capacity for the embodiment of spirit is its capacity for Constant Presence, its abiding devotion to the nourishing of life.

The Phoenix is born in the cinnabar cave, the *dan tian*[5] 丹田 cinnabar field—the depths of the Earth, which also signifies the area of the lower belly in our bodies. The connection between the birthplace of the Phoenix and cinnabar, the metal so highly prized by Taoist alchemists, tells us that there is something about the nature of the Phoenix that is central to alchemical processes. The ancient texts explain that it is from its womb deep in the Earth that the Phoenix produces the essence of Fire, the fuel of the furnace of transformation.

The Phoenix is not a normal bird. Its magic is that it can assimilate and integrate all nature of things and fuel all nature of processes. It can eat every kind of bamboo. It can drink every kind of wine. It can sing every tone. It has a part of every animal within it: head like a chicken, neck like a swan, back like a snake, tail like a fish and wings made of ivory horns.

Most importantly, the Phoenix expresses every virtue through its own being:

- *shun* 順 the character for smooth flowing in the right direction marks its wings

- *zheng* 正 the character for righteousness is on its back

- *xin* 信 the character for faithfulness, trust and integrity is on its belly

- *ren* 仁 the character for loving kindness and benevolence is on its breast

- *de* 德 the character for virtue and authentic Heart-centered being on its head leads the way to Tao.

When the Phoenix is ready, it rises out of its cave with huge transformative power. This heavy bird that carries all aspects of the world within it is born with the capacity for flight. Flying is not easy, and yet its potent strength and strong intention allow the Phoenix to lift off the ground and touch the Heavens. It is said that if this bird starts to fly, all the others will follow. It is also said that when we see the Phoenix in the sky, we know that a good Emperor is ascending to the throne.

The Phoenix reminds us that the Earth is responsible not only for the transformation of food but also for transforming, integrating and assimilating every influence that comes into us from the outside. The Earth, like the Phoenix, can hold it all.

Like the Spleen, the Phoenix must be able to take in but also process, direct and move. It must descend but also ascend. Without this capacity to rise and fall and rise again, there can be no growing, no saving, no storing, no using, no transforming and no nourishing of life.

The Phoenix reminds us that the crucial significance of the Earth, the celestial pivot, is its ability to harmonize the energies of Above and Below. In our own lives, the Phoenix is the connecting link between our original nature, our Tao, and the lives we live each day.

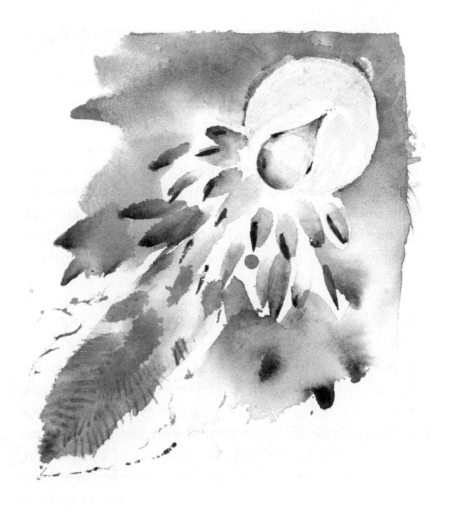

THE PHOENIX

Archetype: The Divine Mother

The essence of the Earth Element is expressed by the archetype of the Divine Mother. Throughout space and time, humans have associated the nurturing, sustaining, protecting aspects of the personal mother with the Earth herself, as well as with the embodied aspect of the Divine. This archetype resides in the matrix of our flesh, our sense memory and our dreams.

It is related to our earliest experiences of embodiment, security, nurturance and compassion.

Through our relationship with the Earth Element, we gain access to the formative potency of the cosmos, to the maker of the myriad beings, the archetypal energy of the Divine Mother. This archetype is associated with generosity, fertility and abundance, with gardens, fields, valleys and hills. Stones warmed by the sun. Apple trees weighed down with fruit. Caverns and caves that open into dark enclosures. Female animals—the cow for her life-giving milk, the pig for her many breasts, the bear for her fierce protectiveness of her cubs.

Whatever nourishes and sustains us comes under her jurisdiction but also whatever stifles, suffocates and pulls us regressively back into our primal longings for safety and ease. Sometimes, she comes bringing the chaotic madness of the great mother goddess of ancient Anatolia, Cybele or Mater Kybeliya, the wild, owl-eyed Mother of the Mountains. Sometimes she comes with the transpersonal love of White Tara, the Buddhist Goddess of Compassion, with innumerable eyes of mercy surrounding her in an aura of golden light. Sometimes she comes with the serenity of Mary, the passionate devotion of Guadalupe, the simplicity of a glass of water, the humble hanging of a coat on a hook on the back of a door or a warm, familiar hand reaching back through time to support us.

The Mother Goddess comes and goes in every healing environment whether we acknowledge her or not. The treatment room becomes a *temenos*—a sacred space—when we consciously acknowledge and invite the Mother in to support treatment. It is not necessary to state this intention out loud in words but rather to make space for the Mother in our body, our imagination, our intention, our *yi*. Our work is to see her "imaginally"—her ravaging hunger, her fertility, her unlimited kindness, her capacity to transform structures and her deep commitment to the unfolding and nourishing of life.

Alchemy: Virtuality

Blazoned on the head of the Phoenix, we find the Chinese character *de*—virtuality:

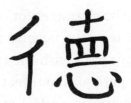

DE - VIRTUE

The character is a complex composite formed by the radical for *chi* 彳 footstep on the left and *zhi* 直 straight over *xin* 心 Heart on the right.

The character for *zhi* 直 was originally a picture of an eye with a straight line above it pointing toward Heaven:

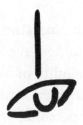

ANCIENT CHARACTER: *ZHI* - STRAIGHT

The ancient character tells us that true virtue comes when we see clearly and in "straight" alignment with Heaven. But the character also reminds us that the straightness that leads to true virtue is not a rigidly prescribed straightness, but rather a pathway that rests on and is tempered by the multidimensional wisdom of the Heart. *De* invites us to move through our life with a unity of eye, Heart and mind. This requires us to open to a special kind of sight, a sight that perceives the intelligence of the Divine here and now in the natural world and that recognizes the connection between our own and this far more expansive intelligence.

Most importantly, the character for "footstep" on the left reminds us that *de*—the virtue beyond all virtues—requires not only that we see our path with the eyes of the Heart but also that we walk this path with our feet on the ground, that we make it true—effective, practical and real! Philosopher and mystic Alan Watts describes *de* as:

> [T]he realization or expression of Tao in actual living...not virtue in the sense of moral rectitude...rather as we speak of the healing virtues of a plant, having the connotation of power or even magic, when magic refers to wonderful and felicitous events which come about spontaneously... possession of a force or power.[6]

Watts goes on to say that this kind of virtue creates space for synchronicities, the impossible coincidences that arise when we open to the possibility of a non-linear life, a way of living that forms out of its own innate *entelechy* rather than the manipulation of the personal will. Virtue in this sense aligns us with Tao, with the mystery and strangeness of the cosmos. It allows us to ride the wind, walk the Earth, drink the dew, enter the water without a ripple and take each day as it comes rather than as we wish it would be.

The Taoist philosopher and poet Chuang Tzu alludes to the importance of strangeness and even weirdness if we are living from a place of *de*.[7] He praises with delight the virtue of the different, of the mysterious workings of the world, of the hunchback and the gnarled and crooked pine tree. He speaks of a particularly useless tree called a *shu*. The trunk of this tree is too gnarled and bumpy to be measured for boards, its branches too twisty for any kind of carpentry. This big tree is worthless per ordinary standards and so it will never be chopped down with an axe for building or any other so-called useful purpose. Rather, it will be left alone to thrive in its own way in the forest. One day, Chuang Tzu suggests, you might come upon this ancient gnarled giant "in the field of Broad and Boundless"[8] and lie down by its side to relax for a while and dream.

The special strangeness of *de* arises from the fullest possible acceptance of my own unique embodiment. It arises from the mingling of the upper and lower spirits in me, the mingling of yang and yin, conscious and unconscious and the powerful buffing and shining of the gold of the *shen* when it descends to Earth and hits the constricting challenges of matter and form.

This virtue *de* is not a limitation but an expansion of possibility. In Chuang Tzu's words, it allows us to "embrace the ten thousand things and roll them into one" rather than wearing ourselves "out over the affairs of the world...though flood waters pile up to the sky, he will not drown."[9]

Earth Spirit Points

Stomach 8 - Head Tied - *Tou Wei*

頭維

Tangled in my thoughts,
I almost missed the firefly's goodbye
in the late-night leaves.

A day so full, my head spins. The garden is bursting with gleaming, plump vegetables clamoring to be eaten and processed, monarch butterflies hatching from their chrysalises and fluttering wildly about the Mexican sunflowers, hedges vibrating with the humming of cicadas and singing of birds. So much to do, to gather, to prepare. And all the while, the honeyed, golden, mid-September sun dripping with sweetness, beckoning me out of my chattering mind, away from my desk, out the door to savor these fleeting moments of glorious late summer sunshine.

Yet, in the midst of the buzz of activity, there is also a release, a returning to rest in the mellow, drifting currents of time, moments to appreciate and take pleasure in the fruits of our labor.

Stomach 8 - Head Tied - *Tou Wei* 頭維 is a point that unknots the tangles of the mind, that cuts a clear path through the "too much" of the material world and frees us to remember the ease of late summer and come present to the delight, gracious acceptance, abundance, comfort and surprising poignancy of the Earth Element.

This point brings us back to the body and to the authentic needs of the self. It releases us from the endless tugging and chatter of thought, the excess cogitation and wheel-spinning that is the less-than-optimal expression of the *yi*. It invites us back from worry and confusion to a clear view of the actual task at hand.

The point name is made up of two characters: *tou* 頭 head, leading or first, and *wei* 维, meaning difficult, joined, tied or fishnet, as well as saved from damage.

We find *tou* 首 head embedded as a radical in the character Tao 道 the Way. This reinforces the spiritual significance for the ancient Taoists of the head as a guiding principle in the organizing of a purposeful life. And yet the character for Tao also reminds us that *tou* 首 the head must be tethered to 辶 the foot, the lower body and the Earth if we are to find our true path through life.

The complex cluster of meanings associated with the graphic *wei* 维 points to the ambiguous nature of the thinking mind. On the one hand, the character refers to the mind's capacity to lead and organize, to help us to make important connections, weave together the various aspects of our world and gather up and store our nourishing ideas. Yet it does not neglect the difficulties, challenges, entrapments and tangles that result from the excess cogitation and overthinking that afflicts an unbalanced Earth Element.

Looking more closely at the character *wei* 维, on the left side, we find *si* 纟, the radical for silk thread. On the right, we see the phonetic *zhui* 隹, an ancient drawing of a bird, sometimes described as a dove but also graphically and phonetically related to *zhu jiao* 朱 鷦, the little Red Bird of the Heart. Hidden within the point name is a clue to the resolution of the contradiction embedded in the graphic. In order to access the devotion, Heart-centered intention and fertile receptivity that are the true expression of a healthy *yi*, we must restore the connection between our Hearts and our mind. By bringing the *yi* back to its nest in the *xin* 心 the Heart, the Head Tied - *Tou Wei* point frees the Red Bird that has been trapped in the net of our tangled thoughts and invites it to settle back down into the nest of the Heart. In this way, our thoughts are free to return to an embodied connection to the immediate present, the mystery, wisdom and beauty of the world around us.

Suggested Essential Oil: Tangerine

Like the bitter orange peel that is used in many Chinese herbal formulas to transform dampness and move qi, tangerine essential oil can be used to support and enliven the energy of the Earth Element. A drop of tangerine on Head Tied - *Tou Wei* is like a spark of golden light. It is a wake-up call for a sleepy brain or a cobweb-filled mind. Tangerine's tangy, vibrant aroma cuts through the stagnancy, bogginess, self-complacency and excess excitation that are the pathological expressions of weak Earth and brings us back to an alert, receptive and mindful presence.

By moving qi, transforming dampness and activating the energies of the *yi*, tangerine oil has the capacity to liberate the spirit and help us to receive the nourishing energies of the world around us. It invites us to be present to the delights of what is here today rather than worrying about the problems that may come tomorrow.

Stomach 12 - Broken Bowl - *Que Pen*
缺盆

What remains as the tide
recedes with the moon, is this breeze
between my fingers.

Looking out over the cove as the tide recedes, I feel my Heart crack open. I long to hold on to the glory of this day. Yet I can no more stop the sun from setting earlier and the nights growing cooler than I can stop this water rushing between the rocks on its way back to the sea. What is asked of me now is presence, acceptance and gratitude for the rhythmic give and take of life, for the transformation of the heat and light of summer into the bounty and generosity of late summer.

This point always reminds me of Sharon, a young mother who came to me soon after the birth of her first child complaining of lethargy, depression and postpartum fatigue. Sharon was exhausted all the time and having trouble digesting food. She was weepy and overwhelmed by day and restless and worried at night. Despite the fact that she had been longing to give birth to a child, her exhaustion and emotional lability made it impossible for her to receive pleasure from her baby.

It was clear to me that one of the main causes of Sharon's exhaustion was lack of nourishment. But her lack of nourishment came not only from her inability to digest food but also from an inability to emotionally digest the profound transformational experience of birth. She could not digest her experience and thus was unable to reap the harvest of her "labor." The joy of motherhood was unavailable to her. One of the most important and beautiful experiences of her life was passing her by, unsavored and undigested, exhausting her every bit as much as her inability to assimilate the food she was eating.

In addition to stimulating the acupuncture points along the Stomach and Spleen meridians, which I knew would help give Sharon the increased levels of energy she was seeking, I decided to look for a point that would touch Sharon at a deeper level. The point I chose was Stomach 12 - Broken

Bowl - *Que Pen* 缺盆. When I shared the translated name of this point with Sharon, she was very moved. She said that a broken bowl described her state of being perfectly—a bowl that could no longer hold things in. All her energy was draining through the cracks. Her brain couldn't retain ideas and her body couldn't hold on to the nourishment of the food she ate. She was unable to contain the experience of motherhood and thus was unable to derive pleasure and delight from it.

The name of this point contains within it a clustering of images, metaphors and meaning. *Que* 缺 means empty, vacant, imperfect or defective. *Pen* 盆 refers to a basin or bowl. On one level, the name reflects the anatomical location of the point. There is a dip or bowl that forms in the body just above the center of the clavicle where this point is found. The bone of the clavicle itself resembles the broken rim of a basin. But this point name has other levels of meaning. The point is located on the Stomach meridian. The Stomach has to do with the holding of food during the initial processes of digestion. Digestion begins in the Stomach as a kind of alchemical cooking or heating of the food. Thus, the Stomach's function is like the function of a bowl. When there is disharmony in the body, the Stomach, like a bowl that is broken, cannot hold the food so that it can be cooked and prepared for assimilation. It cannot properly perform its functions.

There is also a spiritual resonance to this point name that transcends culture. Since the earliest times, people have made bowls out of clay for cooking and eating and crocks and urns for ritual purposes. Women especially were involved in the task of pottery making. Bowls, at an unconscious or "primitive" level, remind us of the maternal bowl, the uterus where new life "cooks" until it is ready, the sacred cauldron where new life is formed. The bowl of the uterus "cracks" like Pan Gu's egg to allow the infant to emerge into the world.[10] In the cracking of the bowl, the One becomes Two, and a new consciousness is born.

For my patient, the wisdom of Broken Bowl - *Que Pen* was already in her as a kind of symbolic, embodied knowing. She had undergone the powerful initiation of giving birth. She herself had become the alchemical vessel in which life cooked. She had been cracked open by the forces of nature in order to bring new life into the world. Yet she did not have the wisdom and containment of a culture with an embodied language to help her reintegrate after this overwhelmingly powerful experience. Like so many women in the West, she was left in a limbo state of postpartum fatigue and disorientation with no way to make the next step into mature womanhood. She needed to make a new connection back to herself and to a meaningful cosmic environment in order to heal. Through the thousands of years of embodied wisdom contained in two simple words, "broken bowl," she was able to make certain connections that helped her mend not just her body but also her soul.

Later, after her treatment had progressed, we came back to the same point. As her condition improved, she spoke about the broken bowl in another way. The broken bowl became like a woman who had given birth; who, through being "broken open," had given birth not only to a child but also to a transformed, more mature self, a woman who could hold things in a new way. The fact that she was no longer "perfect," that she was broken, could be grieved but also celebrated.

The broken bowl became symbolic of her relationship with her own mother, who had not given her the containment and nurturance she needed. Accepting the crack in herself eventually led to an acceptance of the crack in her relationship with her mother. She came to realize that although her relationship with her mother was imperfect, it could still offer her a certain amount of support. This realization freed the mother in Sharon to come to life. It allowed her to be an imperfect, human, creative woman, a vital source of aliveness to herself and her child. She found that giving up being "perfect" and unbroken made room for her new self. This self was able to accept the processes of growth and change that are part of the harvesting of life's experiences.

Suggested Essential Oil: Vetiver

Vetiver is a moist, heavy, calming, nourishing, stabilizing and very fragrant oil that fortifies the Stomach and Spleen. It is useful in cases of deficient Spleen qi and blood, poor appetite and poor absorption of nutrients. It tonifies and calms the nervous system so it can be called on in cases of anxiety, depression, postpartum depression, hyperactive mind, insomnia, insecurity, mental and physical exhaustion and for undernourished perfectionists and perseverating thinkers who are out of touch with their body. It relaxes and cools an overheated mind and brings with it Mother Earth's calm, yin, nurturing strength. When a drop is applied to Broken Bowl - *Que Pen*, this viscous, rich oil begins to reweave fragments and fill in cracks in our souls so that we can contain and hold the psychological and spiritual nutrients we need in order to restore our being and manifest our Tao.

Stomach 25 - Celestial Pivot - *Tian Shu*
天樞

At summer's end, I watch
mackerel clouds paint floating fish
on the sun-lit waves.

As the high Fire of Summer diminishes in mid-August, a more mellow, stable and generous light infuses the atmosphere. A soft, sweet warmth envelops me, like the reliable devotion that can come after wild passion.

Sitting at the edge of a rocky cliff, looking out over the sea toward the horizon line, I view the great rotunda of Earth and Heaven. I watch the shapes of clouds reflected in the water and the color of water reflected in the sky. On this day of celestial turning, at the beginning of the season of harvest, I feel my own place at the center-point between Above and Below, secure in the harmony of all things.

On one level, the name of this point, Stomach 25 - Celestial Pivot - *Tian Shu* 天樞, refers to its physical location at the exact midline of the body. On a more subtle body level, Celestial Pivot - *Tian Shu* marks the intersection of the upper and lower spirits, the place where sun meets shadow, where Heavenly and Earthly qi unite, the horizon line—the domain of the *yi* spirit—where celestial influences become visible in material form.

Bilaterally, the point brackets the umbilicus, the place where we connect in utero to the stream of maternal nourishment. In this way, Celestial Pivot - *Tian Shu* returns us to our source and anchors our life in the matrix of the Earth Mother who has nurtured us from our beginning.

The point is intimately connected to the *yi*, the spirit of Earth. The *yi* endows us with intention and the capacity to bring the implicit possibilities of the yang upper spirits—the *shen* and *hun*—into yin manifest form. The *yi* holds the center. It allows us to stay steady amid the uncertainties and vicissitudes of embodied existence. Just as the Stomach is in charge of digesting physical food and transforming it into physical muscle, the *yi* is charged with digesting experience and transforming it into psychic muscle. A healthy *yi* allows us "to do," to set a clear intention, complete the projects we begin and engender real change in a physical form.

While this point has many physical-level indications including persistent diarrhea, edema, nausea and menstrual disorders, it also has other important psycho-spiritual effects. It is key to the regulation and tonification of the *yi*. It helps to restore harmony between Above and Below and communication between the upper and lower spirits. But most of all, it brings us back to our own authentic nature, our own steady sense of self. It helps to keep us stable in the midst of change and trust the sacredness of our own body knowing.

Suggested Flower Essence: Cerato

Cerato is a flower essence that supports us in listening to our own inner knowledge. It helps us cultivate an enlivened relationship to our authentic inner voice so that we can attend to the counsel of others without losing connection to the self. How do we know the "right thing to do," the right next step that will move us further along the path of our Tao, since there is no one right Way for all? As I take in the support of this sky-blue, five-petaled flower, I am called to listen more deeply to my own deep body knowing, my own "felt sense," the inner voice that can tell me what is true and right for me. Cerato flower essence connects me to my instinctual nature, bringing with it grounded, calm confidence in my own being. It opens us without force yet with great determination to our own inner wisdom.

The clarity of this sky-blue flower reminds me of how I feel when I am truly in touch with my own center so that Heaven and Earth align in me. In particular, it supports me in paying attention to the somatic murmurs of my breath, my "gut," my muscles and my bones and helps me to know what I want and need here on Earth and what is being asked of me by Heaven.

Stomach 40 - Abundant Splendor - *Feng Long*
豐隆

At one with the buzz
of the honeybees, I sip the last
sweet nectar of the sun.

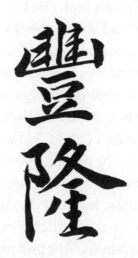

Earth season arrives, expected but still taking my body by surprise. I walk out into the cooler garden and I feel a heaviness come over me. The sunflowers can barely hold up their dark heads. The squash have swollen overnight to inedible sizes. The ghosts of Autumn are still hidden behind the curtain of the green world but I hear their preparations, the rustling of their skirts and jackets as they stretch and yawn in their underworld beds and the snapping of twigs as they pick the dry dirt from underneath their fingernails.

There is something unbearable about how quickly summer ends. I am not ready. I need a pause, an interval between the untempered joyous exuberance of July and the poignant loss of November. I am not ready to go down and yet there is not enough lightness left to lift me. But then I remember the seeds.

The seeds I have promised to gather for friends are ready now, waiting in perfect equilibrium at the tips of the stems and branches, tucked into the curled fists of the dry Queen Anne's Lace, hunkered down in the husks of the mallow, rattling their tiny teeth in the poppy pods. I go in for bottles, bags and baskets and begin collecting. As I tear open the husks and pods and fists, there is an explosion— not only seeds but an infinitude of life: feasting fleas, delicate white spiders, nasty snapping earwigs and segmented green caterpillars emerge, sleepy and sated yet lively.

Right here, right now, at the middle of the Wheel, at the center of the seasons, at the meeting point of the darkness and the light, nature exudes a reckless delight in the abundance of it all—even with autumn, loss and death around the corners, so much abundance, so much life to celebrate! As we read in the *I Ching*, Hexagram 55 - Abundance - *Feng*, "To bring about a time of abundance, a union of clarity and energetic movement is needed."[11]

Stomach 40 - Abundant Splendor - *Feng Long* 豐隆 is a point that gathers up the spirit of Late Summer and distributes it through our being. You find this point waiting patiently for touch, approximately one inch lateral to the anterior crest of the tibia, midway between the ankle and the knee crease. It will work to transform phlegm, bring clarity to the Heart and mind, and endow us with the capacity for measured and potent action. I call on its wisdom when people feel overwhelmed by too much goodness and need support in knowing how and when to receive, digest and distribute the bounty of their own life. When our "plate is too full" and yet there is much to be grateful for, we can turn to Abundant

Splendor - *Feng Long* to help us remember how to celebrate the harvest.

Stomach 44 - Inner Courtyard - *Nei Ting*

內庭

At the garden gate,
my old friend waits, while I pick
her fragrant catnip leaves.

Then, in early September, there is a day that whispers secrets in my ear, a day when I need to listen carefully in order not to miss the messages and melodies of this season. At the edges of the woods, I discover fantastically shaped mushrooms that have sprung up overnight from the damp lawn, moss and pine needles: dirty white puffballs, carbon-black fringed inky caps and shaggy manes, crimson-topped amanitas, sulfur-yellow chicken of the woods. As I pass the stand of black cohosh, honeybees erupt in buzzing clouds from the towering flower spikes, hauling off foraged clumps of pollen on their hind legs. And as I stop to watch the bees fly back to their hive, I hear a single cricket resume his sad, lonely love song from under the tin watering can.

Although the sunflowers are still bright and a bit over-blown and the cucumbers in the garden still clamor enthusiastically over the embankment, I can feel that the summer festivities are winding down, that despite the full display of flowers and fruit, everything has already begun to draw inward. The heat and yang activity of the previous months are dwindling, sinking, drooping and dropping down into the soil to be sequestered and stored in the seeds and roots of plants and trees until next spring.

There is an intimacy to the sunlight as it touches my bare feet in the grass, a new shy quiet to the morning. Making my way down to the vegetable garden to check up on the lettuce and kale, I turn to see my cat, Professor, following me silently along the path, her whiskered face gazing quizzically back at me from an inscrutable mystery, the secret language of the inner world of nature that is far, far older than words.

Stomach 44 - Inner Courtyard - *Nei Ting* 內庭 is a point that touches us at the level of this mystery. The character *nei* 內 means "inside"—a secret place, the interior of a house or an inner chamber. The design of the graphic itself can be viewed as an archetypal reference to the opening to a woman's pelvis and reinforces the use of the word to refer to one's wife or her relatives who traditionally lived in the hidden, inner spaces of the home. At times, *nei* is also used to describe a kind of wisdom that is hidden or esoteric such as the *nei dan*, the inner esoteric aspect of alchemy, as opposed to outer or common knowledge.

The character is made up of two parts. The lower part, the radical that means "to enter," looks something like the doorway to a tent or hut, and also like the little "V" between the second and third toe where this point is located. Enclosing *ru* 入 is an ancient graphic 冂, which was used to depict an area beyond the border of a known territory, a distant or empty space or void, an unknown place. The character *ting* 庭 is a picture of a house 广 covering 壬, a monarch, master or host, and the radical 廴 meaning journey.

The etymology of the point name reinforces our understanding of the intimacy and secret, esoteric nature of this point. In the poem "The Ode to the Jade Dragon," attributed to the 12th-century Taoist sage and acupuncturist Ma Danyang (see note 20 on page 286), Inner Courtyard - *Nei*

Ting is included in the list of Danyang's Twelve Heavenly Star Points.[12]

On a physical level, we recognize that, as the Water point on the Stomach meridian, Inner Courtyard - *Nei Ting* calls up the special qualities and capacities of Water—hiddenness, calm, depth, renewal and smooth flow—that are sequestered in the Earth. Danyang describes the power of this point to drain heat from the interior, specifically the Stomach channel, harmonize the intestines, stimulate the appetite, alleviate the pain of a toothache, clear skin rashes and staunch a bloody nose. He also emphasizes the psycho-emotional actions of the point. He speaks in particular of its ability to restore the righteous flow of qi and spread life-giving warmth back from the core of the body to the limbs when there are deathly cold hands and feet due to acute emotional or physical shock.[13]

However, through a closer reading of the Ode, we discover that the unique spirit of this point is embedded in the etymology of the point name. Not only is the point said to calm the *shen* but Danyang also speaks of its ability to soothe the spirit when one is overwhelmed by noise or in a depressive state with a desire for silence, particularly when there is a "hatred of loud voices" and disturbing activity in the outer world. We turn to this point when a person needs the healing seclusion and quiet of the interior or when the medicine needed is found deep within the body or within a secret, cloistered space. Inner Courtyard - *Nei Ting* takes us on a journey to this space of calm and meditation, a place away from the world of words and chatter, a place where we can go to appreciate the nourishment of the Earth, the healing warmth of the late summer sunlight and the quiet peace of the inner gardens of the embodied soul. Indeed, Danyang tells us that "a needle here means true awakening."[14]

Suggested Needle Technique

In the second section of the Ode, instructions are given for the activation of the Heavenly Star Points. Although the points are not themselves secret, the activating of their deeper mysterious functions requires inner work and self-cultivation on the part of the practitioner. The meditation offered by Danyang is to imagine that needling these points is like "pouring hot water on snow."[15] When I reflect on this image as I open the spirit level of Inner Courtyard - *Nei Ting* with a needle, there is no great, overt effort, yet great change is effected at the level of how a person feels inside. In needling this point, I must maintain an intimate connection to myself, my patient and the needle between my fingers. I bring the intention of touching a deeply introverted spirit with gentle kindness, offering a very special kind of nourishment to the animal soul: the medicine of wordless presence.

Spleen 3 - Supreme White - *Tai Bai*

太白

On the high branches
of the pine, an osprey preens
white feathers in the sun.

On the morning of the autumn equinox, I watch the sun make its way up from the eastern horizon. As the equator reaches its momentary equilibrium and then tips northward, I notice a new quality of substance, weight and majesty to the sun's ascent. Rather than the buoyant lift of summer, there is an upward climb that now takes effort. The sunlight feels denser, more honeyed and, in some way, more precious. The warmth is measured; aged, mellowed and layered like wine by the passage of time. The glory, when the golden sun at last tips over the tops of the trees, is breathtaking.

Spleen 3 - Supreme White - *Tai Bai* 太白 is the source and the Earth within the Earth point on the Spleen meridian. It is a point that epitomizes the power and the medicine of Earth and Late Summer. As source, it is adaptogenic. It knows what is needed. It lifts what is heavy, astringes what is damp, tonifies deficiency and clears excess. It brings the digesting, nourishing and transporting aspects of the Earth into balance and harmony.

The point name is made up of the character *tai* 太 great and *bai* 白 white but also clear and pure. *Bai* is a picture of the sun with a *pie dian* or left-curving dash stroke at the top. The character is a graphic depiction of a ray of light pointing upward as the sun rises in the sky. The name reinforces my understanding that this is a point with great power: the power to lift and to rise, to lighten, clarify and move. When I touch this point, I access a rich source of qi that rises up to nourish and energize my entire being while, at the same time, stabilizing and grounding me. In addition, on the spirit level, I discover the greatness of this point in its ability to restore my delight and appetite for life and to support the feeling of abundance and generosity that is so much a part of the Earth's intrinsic nature.

I am also intrigued by the connection between the point name and *Tai Bai Xing* 太白星 Great White Star, the Chinese name for the planet Venus. The connection between the point name and the planet deepens my understanding of the spirit of the point. Throughout time and across cultures, the bright light of Venus that shines just before sunrise on the eastern horizon and shimmers just after sunset in the western sky has been associated with beauty, the mystery of rising light and falling darkness, along with a particular kind of feminine wisdom and illuminating love. The crucial mother–child connection between Earth and Metal is highlighted not only by the inclusion of Metal's white color in the point name but also by the association with Venus, the "white star" that the Chinese specifically associated with the western direction and the Metal Element. From the clues embedded in the point name, I realize that I can turn to this point when I feel the need to restore the connection between mother, Earth, and child, Metal.

Classic texts suggest Supreme White - *Tai Bai* when excess Earth and deficient Metal result in physical symptoms such as loose stools, diarrhea and constipation due to insufficient Spleen qi to activate and move the bowels. However, on a spirit level, I also consider Supreme White - *Tai Bai* when Metal is calling for Earth's support in order to restore its brightness and shine. Like a mother's love for her child, the great shining light of this point helps a person who is feeling lost, empty and uninspired to rise up above the weight of despair, renew a sense of personal preciousness, clarify purpose and open their wings once again to the steadfast, resilient and generous light of the late summer morning sun.

Suggested Treatment: Amber with Rice Grain Moxa

Amber gemstones form from the sticky resin of ancient evergreen trees that have fossilized and crystallized over millennia. The golden light that emanates from the depth of the stone has been considered a mystery since Neolithic times. Pieces of carved amber have been found alongside the bones of the dead in cave burials dating back to 10,000 BCE. Archetypally, the stone is associated with sunlight and honey and its capacity to store and restore is visible in the perfectly preserved skeletons of insects that are often found as inclusions trapped inside the translucent mineralized resin.

Supreme White - *Tai Bai* is highly responsive to the warmth, weight and light of amber resin oil. While pure amber essence oil is extremely expensive, even a minute amount diluted in carrier oil is sufficient to activate the magic and medicine of the point. If the oil or resin is unavailable, touching the point with the gemstone is also highly effective. Application of the oil or gemstone followed by three to five rice grain moxa will enhance the nourishing, activating, lifting, grounding and warming capacities of the point and help a person to know both their own strength and their own sweetness.

Spleen 5 - Merchant Mound - *Shang Qiu*
商丘

Too many beans to pick!
Instead I sit and sip green tea
in the morning rain.

As the Late Summer season progresses toward Autumn, the early exuberance of the harvest bogs down. There is just too much matter to deal with. The compost overflows its bin. The zucchini plants, which have grown to unmanageable proportions, continue to pump out food well after the appetite for summer squash has faded. The remaining monarch caterpillars grow in size but do not transform as they chew listlessly at the remaining milkweed leaves. There is still enough yang heat and light for growth and production to continue but not enough yang qi to transform, distribute and move all the yin accumulations along.

Standard modern acupuncture texts emphasize the tendency for the Spleen to become deficient. For example, in *A Manual of Acupuncture*, we read, "The Spleen, dominating the ceaseless yang functions of transportation and transformation, easily becomes deficient in qi and yang, and therefore most of its patterns of disharmony involve deficiency."[16] And yet, in the treatment room, I often see symptoms in my Earth patients that appear more like excess than deficiency, more like what I feel and what I see in the garden at the end of the harvest: over-production, over-accumulation, too much to think about, too much to do, too much to process. Of course, the underlying issue is almost always about "not enough"—not enough time, not enough energy, not enough yang qi left to move it all along. Adding more of anything to an already full belly, an overflowing compost bin or a damp and phlegm-filled Spleen only adds to the back-up and does nothing to support the process of transformation. This is when I call on the wisdom of Metal within the Earth, the wisdom of Spleen 5 - Merchant Mound - *Shang Qiu* 商丘.

The Metal point on the Spleen meridian, Merchant Mound - *Shang Qiu* has the capacity to support the clearing out and letting go of accumulations but also the capacity to distill out the preciousness and perceive what is valuable in the food, experiences and impressions we take in. Taking a closer look at the point name, we find the character *shang* 商, meaning discuss, merchant or businessperson (as well as the second note of the pentatonic scale, which is associated with the Metal Element). The character is made up of two parts: *yan* 言 a picture of a mouth playing music, meaning speech or language, and *nei* 内, referring to what is in the interior. *Shang* points to the necessity of bringing out what is within in order to achieve an honorable transaction. The righteous merchant is one who speaks from her interiority and in this way makes a successful business dealing. She promotes the exchange of commodities and products for money and energy. In the process of the transactions, she eliminates accumulations and moves things along!

The character *qiu* 丘 refers to a mound, grave or hill. I see the various interpretations of the character as an allusion to the paradox of the Earth—a place of growth, life potential, nourishment and riches, but also of stagnation, burial and death. What is contained within the mound is important but even more crucial is the question of how I make use of it.

For me, the underlying message of this curious point name is that the paradox of the Spleen—deficiency of yang that leads to an excess of yin—can be resolved through a skillful transaction that ultimately leads to an exchange between the Earth and the Metal elements. This means that, on a spirit level, I must make my peace with letting go of what has accumulated, even if that includes a culling or a death, in order to reactivate stagnating transformational processes and maintain the vitality of the *sheng* cycle—the Wheel of Life. Sometimes, when my Spleen has gone on overdrive, I have to stop, let go, drink a cup of green tea and surrender to the mystery.

Suggested Essential Oil: Helichrysum

This essential oil is distilled from the blossoms of the aromatic shrub known as strawflower. The flowers are easily dried and keep their shape and color over winter. For this reason, the plant is also often referred to as "Immortelle" or "Everlasting." The oil, which is distilled from the blossoms, has a potent and unique aroma, a dusty, sharp and golden scent that for me is strongly reminiscent of the chrysanthemums of late summer and the drying leaves of early autumn. The aroma brings together the sweetness of the Earth and the pungent dryness of Metal.

Helichrysum oil has strong qi-moving, anti-inflammatory and anti-coagulating properties. It can be used as a first-aid treatment for bruising and head and muscle aches and is often used in small amounts in combination with carrier oils to heal and refine the skin and reduce the appearance of wrinkles. However, when used in accompaniment with a needle on Merchant Mound - *Shang Qiu*, its spirit-level action has both a calming, dispersing and an invigorating, tonifying effect. When I am blocked in my ability to open to my deep resources, my faith and my willingness to surrender, this oil dislodges impediments and doubts and awakens my soul to the possibility of letting go in order to receive a death that is also a renewal.

Spleen 8 - Earth Motivator - *Di Ji*

也機

Morning glories climb
over the garden gate... just in time
to greet the sunflowers.

The day breaks with a cloudless sky the color of blue morning glories. The breeze has freshened and lightly bites my skin as I step outside. Looking up, I see three monarchs flying southwest on the updrafts, flying with a meandering but unhesitating purpose in the direction of the light.

There is a wake-up call in the atmosphere, an invigorating tingle, an imperative toward manifestation, fulfillment, harvest. All of nature seems to be saying, "Now!" "Get going!" It's time to move, time to get things done.

Spleen 8 - Earth Motivator - *Di Ji* 也機 is a point that resonates with this kind of late summer morning. It is the antidote to the Earth's problematic tendency toward lethargy, apathy, bloating, dampness, stagnation, procrastination and self-pity. The point enlivens the Earth's healthy appetite for life and supports its authentic capacity to actively build muscularity rather than passively consume resources.

The character *di* 地 means earth—land, soil, fields—but also can be used to indicate a territory or place at some distance away. There is an implied potency, movement and directionality to this character that is not present in the character *tu* 土 Earth when used on its own. *Ji* 機 is made of the radical *mu* 木 Wood and the phonetic *ji* 幾, meaning some or "how many?" *Ji* 機 is used to mean a machine or, in modern times, an airplane, but also to indicate a critical moment, a crucial point in a process.

The simplest way to understand the spirit of this point from a first glimpse at the etymology of the point name is to say that it refers to the activating capacity of the Earth Element, its ability to use resources (*mu* 木 Wood) to build and nourish the muscle power or inner machinery that allows us to move and to make things real in the outer world. But a deeper understanding comes when we recall the presence of the radical *ji* 機 in the Chinese word *wei ji* 危機 crisis, which, for the Chinese, also implies opportunity. Here we see that *ji* refers to a moment when we are presented with a situation that needs to be dealt with skillfully. The decisions we make, the actions we take and how we use the resources at hand can transform a crisis that looks like a catastrophe into an opportunity that brings tremendous benefits.

Looking more closely at the word *ji* 幾 we find the radical *si* 幺, a silk cocoon with threads, above the radical *shu* 戍 frontier guards. Frontier guard soldiers were given the responsibility of guarding the boundary lands and edges of the known territory. In order to fulfill their assigned function, they had to be absolutely attentive to the finest movements of "silk threads" in the world around them—the infinitesimal changes in the atmosphere, the slightest snapping of a twig or rustle of grass. From these small, nearly imperceptible signs, they had to be able to spring into action without hesitation and to move assertively in the right direction. Acupuncturist and scholar Debra Kaatz enumerates the various levels of meaning contained in the character *ji* as "the causes of changes; the changes of the future; the origin of, the moving power of a machine; secret; cunning; and to seize an opportunity."[17]

Taking all this into account as we approach the spirit of the point Earth Motivator - *Di Ji*, we understand that, at the deepest level, this point opens us to our capacity to notice the tendencies of growth, the small movements that point in the direction of change, and then to assertively grasp opportunities for right action as they arise. It gives us the inner power to resist the pull of doubt and persevere with the job at hand until it is complete. It empowers us to make good use of the resources we have and move forward with *yi*—strong, clear intention—yet with cunning, stealth and close attention to the details. And like late summer sunlight, it energizes our desire to seize the day, to rise up to greet life's challenges with optimistic enthusiasm and to move forward with resilience and grace even when the ground is rough or the territory distant and unknown.

Suggested Essential Oil: Coriander

Coriander seeds have a long history as a medicinal herb. The seeds are used as a digestive tonic in Chinese medicine and a digestive, carminative and nerve tonic in the Western herbal tradition. In addition, coriander has long been regarded as a sacred herb with protective and preserving properties. The seeds have been discovered in the tombs of ancient Egyptian kings and the leaves are used to this day as one of the bitter herbs served at the Passover Seder.

Coriander essential oil supports the Earth Element by transforming phlegm and dampness into functional movement and change. It has an affinity to the Spleen and Stomach and tonifies digestion, assimilation and distribution of nutrients at all levels. Coriander essential oil roots and stabilizes and, at the same time, imbues a feeling of liveliness and spontaneity. It brings clarity of mind, stability of intention and buoyancy of spirit to the Earth Element.

A drop of coriander on this point enlivens our sense of purpose, activates potential and helps to eliminate phlegmatic lethargy. At the same time, it offers a feeling of safety and protection to the spirit as we move forward in our embodied life on Earth, along the unique path of our Tao.

Spleen 9 - Yin Mound Spring - *Yin Ling Quan*
陰 陵 泉

At the pond's moist edge,
a chorus of frogs sings dirges
to the dancing dragonflies.

As late summer days continue to cool and move downward toward the yin, ripening processes slow and moisture accumulates. As the season fulfills its promise of abundance, there is also the danger of a surfeit of supply and this, in turn, can lead to over-accumulation, dampness and stagnancy. What is needed now is a review of our inventory and a reckoning. We are invited to come to terms with the consequences of our actions, to assess our successes and failures and find ways to process, digest and assimilate the fruits of the seeds we sewed earlier in the cycle of life.

When the products of our inspirations, visions, plans and efforts are undigested and hoarded, the harvest stagnates. The fruit rots rather than ripens on the vine. The effect is bloating, sluggishness and resistance, rather than generosity, nourishment, motivation and transformation. As entropy takes over, there is a gradual erosion of the connections between Above and Below, between the enlivening energies of the upper spirits and the manifesting potential of the lower spirits. When the Earth Element—the Stomach and Spleen— hoard rather than disseminate their resources, nutrients and fluids are sequestered. Earth's child, Metal, grows brittle and cold and its grandchild, Water, is deprived of its rich legacy of suppleness, vitality, resilience and courage.

Spleen 9 - Yin Mound Spring - *Yin Ling Quan* 陰 陵 泉 is a point for this impasse that at times may afflict the Earth Element. It opens the flow between the gathering and disseminating capacities of the Earth. It revitalizes the *yi* and infuses the body with the renewing potency of yin moisture. Like a gentle breeze or an iridescent dragonfly that restores light and movement to the sluggish stillness of a brackish point, a needle skillfully inserted into this point enlivens stuck qi *and* draws stagnant moisture and accumulated dampness back into the life cycle.

The middle character of the point name, *ling* 陵 mound, gives us a clue to the deeper meaning of the point. In addition to meaning mound or hill, it also is used to refer to a tomb or mausoleum. It is composed of two radicals: *zhi* 夂 to walk slowly or with difficulty and *lu* 坴 land but also containing the idea of *lu* 圥, a mushroom pushing up from the soil below. The character *ling* 夌 as a whole contains the idea of something vital from down below that pushes up against obstacles, a hill that is difficult to walk across or a place where something that has died or gone down to the underworld is stored. The *quan* 泉 spring that rises up from this underworld place is resourceful, determined, regenerative, enlivening and capable of moving through challenges and obstacles.

Yin Mound Spring - *Yin Ling Quan* is the point that opens the flow channel in you. It connects us to the refreshing enlivening springs of vitality that rise up from our bodies and the Earth. In this way, it supports us in facing the obstacle or impediments that prevent us from moving forward in our lives and gives our souls access to the vitalizing springs that rise up from our bodies and the Earth.

On a physical level, Yin Mound Spring - *Yin Ling Quan* brings movement, buoyancy and flow when there is edema, distension, retention of urine or difficult urination, swelling of the knee and issues with undigested food. On a psycho-emotional level, it transforms self-pity, exhaustion and muddled thinking into empathy, vitality and refreshing new ideas. And on the level of the spirit, we turn to this point when we are unable to digest and assimilate the experiences in order to progress freely into the next stages of our life.

Suggested Flower Essence: Cayenne

A drop of cayenne flower essence on Yin Mound Spring - *Yin Ling Quan* catalyzes change and brings movement to the stagnant places within us. The medicine of the fiery, energetic flower stimulates the body's capacities to face the challenges of change and growth and awakens the soul's capacities to resist procrastination, self-pity and apathy in order to move forward with the journey of our lives.

Spleen 21 - Great Enveloping - *Da Bao*
大包

After the rainstorm,
cormorant hangs her dark wings out
to dry in the sun.

The archetype I most often associate with the Earth Element is the ancient Greek goddess Gaia, the primal, ancestral mother and nurturer of all life. My first acupuncture teacher, J. R. Worsley, writes that as we move from Summer to Late Summer, Fire's "sharing of joy and laughter gives way to a different kind of love, the love of a mother for her children."[18] This love of the Earth is given not only in the form of physical food and emotional care but also in the way that "the Earth as our mother feeds the spirit."[19] When we are fed by the Earth in this way, it is as if we have the love, support and nurturing strength of a good mother. We trust that we will have enough of what we need, not only to survive at a physical level but also to thrive at the level of our soul and our spirit. Through the mother's intrinsic generativity, generosity and stability, we feel that we are held, protected and nurtured and that our spirit has a safe home in our physical body.

However, there is another quality of the mother archetype that I feel is necessary for a complete understanding of the Earth and that is her humility. The word "humility" comes from the Latin root *humilis* meaning low or on the ground and *humus* meaning earth or soil. From this root also comes our word "human" and "humanity." To be human, then, implies a coming from but also a returning to and an honoring of the Earth, the soil, the mother and matrix of matter. To be fully human requires that we accept both the limitations and the great gifts of matter, that we stay right size, that we stay humble and that we take care of and care about the physical domain as the knowable abode of the Divine.

I regard Spleen 21 - Great Enveloping - *Da Bao* 大包 as a spirit point that allows us to access these various qualities of the Earth and empowers us to extend them outward. Great Enveloping - *Da Bao* is the exit point of the Spleen meridian, the point through which we gather up all the energies of the Earth and pass them along, full circle, to nourish the Monarch of the Heart through Heart 1 - Utmost Source - *Ji Quan*. It is a point that puts us in touch with the Earth's capacity to hold, to spread, to freely nourish and to receive as it ends and begins a cycle of growth on the meridian level.

The radical *da* 大 big is used to refer to an adult or elder. It is a picture of a person with arms outstretched wide to the sky, a person coincidentally opening access to the energies of Great Enveloping - *Da Bao* at the sixth (or seventh) intercostal space on the lateral side of the rib cage. *Bao* 包 is a picture of *si* 巳 an embryo wrapped in a *bao* 勹, which represents the maternal womb. From the etymology of the point, we understand that the spirit of this point has something to do with opening to our "bigness" while protecting, holding and nourishing what is small and still coming to life in us. There is a quality of extension but also containment, of reaching out to the world and up to the Heavens while also staying enveloped or encased, of expanding and opening while also protecting and embracing what is vulnerable.

While the widely recognized traditional Chinese medicine applications of this point are limited to pain in the whole body, flaccidity of the joints, cough and chest pain in the lateral costal region,[20] its lesser-known applications make it invaluable. We can open this point when there is a block between the Earth's harvest and the Heart's nourishment leading to blood stagnation and deficiency. On a meridian level, consider needling Great Enveloping - *Da Bao* when there is an obstruction in the flow of qi between the Spleen and Heart meridians on the level of the Chinese clock, resulting in a variety of physical and psycho-emotional symptoms, including a feeling of constraint in the chest, anxiety, exhaustion, depression and heaviness of limbs.

On a spirit level, we turn to this point when we want to open ourselves to the energies of Heaven in a humble and embodied way. We can offer it as a gift to a person who has lost their trust in the safety of their own body or to help heal the wounds of a person who has never known the enveloping, loving support of a good mother.

I touch this point when I am longing to feel the flow of life as it moves through my body, soul and spirit. Like the black cormorant with spread wings, balanced precariously on her stone at the ocean's edge, I humbly open my arms to receive the love, nourishment and harmonizing energies of Gaia, the Earth, through this sacred portal.

Suggested Flower Essence: Mariposa Lily

Mariposa lily is the flower essence to consider when a person has been wounded in their early relationship to their mother or experienced loss relating to the primary nurturing person in their life. When we feel unloved, unsupported and unnourished by the feminine energies and the yin, this beautiful wild lily brings a renewal of trust and faith in the Earth and healing of our connection to the Divine Mother archetype who embraces the entire human family with compassion and nurturing, even if our own mothers have been unable to provide us with what we needed as a child.

A drop of this flower essence on Great Enveloping - *Da Bao* augments the power of the needle and helps us to feel the loving embrace of the mother and the sustaining presence of Gaia at our side.

Metal: Autumn Season

Since the earliest times, metal has held a fascination for human beings. Somehow we know that this element hidden deep beneath the Earth contains the secrets of stars. Metal's crystalline structure and durability, its stillness, its capacity to hold form and value over time, its weight and dignity, its inertness when cold and malleability when sufficiently warmed, its inner luster and ability to reflect light, to shield and protect as well as to penetrate... These qualities teach us about an aspect of our own nature as well as the nature of the world. The Metal Element lives not only in the most basic processes of our bodies—our mineral structure, our skin, our immune system and our breath—but also in our souls.

The Chinese character for Metal is *jin* 金. It is a picture of the character for *tu* 土 Earth covered by a canopy. Under the canopy of the Earth, the two dots represent two nuggets of gold buried deep in the darkness.

In traditional Chinese medicine, the Metal Element is related to the season of Autumn. It represents a time of year when the life force returns to the underworld. It is an expression of qi that is cool, yin, reflective and slow-moving.

We find Metal at the right, yin, low point of the Five Element Wheel. This placement affirms our understanding of its connection to entropy, to the wisdom we find when we rust and decay, when we go down rather than up. Classical texts tell us that "the term metal means restrain."[1] At this point on the Wheel, there is a restriction of growth, a pressure down into the depths. This downward directionality, letting go or exhalation is reflected in autumn's falling leaves and decaying vegetation. As we witness the dwindling of obvious vitality in plants, the slowing down of growth, the emergence of the intrinsic structure of trees and landscape as leaves fall from the branches, we are witnessing the Metal Element moving into ascendancy in the environment.

Kigo words evoke this atmosphere of release and surrender that is Metal's hallmark: last harvest, dwindling light, buried seeds, pumpkins lit with candles, chilly nights with light mists that remind us of ghosts and memories, geese flying south in formation across a steel-gray sky. Metal calls us to the experience of exhalation, letting go, descent, loss and death. But it also invites us to the experience of inhalation, receiving, prayer, inspiration and resurrection. Metal brings us to the immediate and acute realization of the preciousness of the moment, the sacredness of awareness and the understanding that our life is a gift we cannot hold on to.

Vegetative Expression

The vegetative expression of this Element is the decaying plant and the hard, ripened seed that surrenders to the force of gravity as it falls from its husk and is buried beneath the earth. The letting go, rotting and composting that naturally follows this "fall" is part of the transformational potency of the Metal Element. As negentropic life energies dwindle and form disintegrates, the organic structure of the plant breaks down to its base components. Along with the dross left behind, we discover treasure, the fine bits of shining crystals, the inert mineral substrate of life that will support and sustain the building of new organic structures, new life after a time of dying.

Color/Sound/Odor/Emotion

The Color of Metal is White

The *Neijing Suwen* tells us that "White is the color of the West, it pervades the lungs and lays open the nose and retains the essential substance with the lungs."[2] Yet there is something about the whiteness of Metal that goes beyond color to become a kind of shining translucence that hovers above the skin itself. To diagnose the health of the Metal Element, observe the color at the edges of the temples, around the eyes, nose and mouth. Often, this will show up clinically as a kind of shine rather than a color. In describing the variations of white, the *Neijing Suwen* says that "the color of life displayed by the lungs is like the lucky red lining of a white silk robe... when their color is shiny like the grease of pigs they are full of life...when white like dried and withered bones they are without life."[3] In health, we see the shine of spirit hovering above the skin. In disease or imbalance, it expresses as a lackluster dullness. Get to know white by observing the color of white in the world around you, in clouds, snow, birch bark, quartz, feathers and fungus, and look to see how it is reflected in the hues and tones that shine from a person's complexion.

The Sound is Weep

The Metal Element is about letting go and going down, and this is reflected in its sound. The voice may be wispy as if the person is barely there or already leaving. There may be a quality of longing and poignancy and a sense that they are speaking from a distance. The weep may also be heard as a sigh or a thinning out and descending at the end of a sentence. Most markedly, the weep induces a feeling that the chest is constricted and tears are waiting on the other side of the word.

The Odor is Rotten

In balance, the odor of Metal is like humus, well-tended compost, autumn mushrooms or the underside of freshly fallen leaves. However, when there is disease in the Lungs or the Large Intestine is full, this smell changes and can become either metallic, like the smell of a dirty metal garbage can, or unpleasantly rotten, like water-saturated compost that has not been aerated or decaying food.

The Emotion is Grief

In a state of imbalance, the emotion of Metal shows up as rigidity, a clinging to the past, stubborn depression and unrelenting mourning that completely engulfs a person's life and does not shift with the passage of time. However, in health, grief expresses as a willingness to accept the inevitability of loss and the preciousness of each passing moment. At its best, grief shows as a spiritual acceptance and spaciousness that brings peace and mindful presence to everyone it touches.

The Officials

Metal is related to the organs of the Lungs and Large Intestine. On a physical level, these two officials maintain the health of the respiratory and excretory systems. They are in charge of protecting us from pathogenic factors through the integrity of the skin and the immune system. On a mental–emotional level, the main function of these two officials is to support us in letting go of what is obsolete and devitalized to make space to receive what is new, inspiring and enlivening. On the level of the body, the mind and the spirit, their job is to help us self-regulate our internal rhythms in the face of change.

The Lung Official is said to have "the charge of minister and chancellor, from it stem well-regulated rhythms."[4] This function of rhythmic regulation relates to the respiratory function of the Lungs that affects all the rhythms of the body and the mind, including the heart rate, blood flow, peristalsis and cranial rhythms. In fact, the breath is the only direct link between the *hun* and the upper spirits and the *po* and the lower spirits. The breath is the only way we can consciously influence the unfolding of unconscious autonomic processes.

The Large Intestine Official is described in the classical texts as the official "in charge of the roadways and transmissions. Changes and transformations proceed from there."[5] J. R. Worsley speaks of it as "the Dust Bin Collector, the Drainer of the Dregs."[6] This official disposes of and casts away all the waste and rubbish within us—not only on a physical level but on an emotional and spiritual level as well. The Large Intestine Official is like the station master who encourages us to leave behind the heavy suitcases full of old books and clothing and extraneous "stuff" so that we can step on to the train of our life, make room for what we need for our journey and move more lightly forward.

Po: The Spirit of Metal

The spirit of the Metal Element is *po* 魄, which is translated as vegetative or animal soul. The *Neijing Suwen* tells us that Metal is related to the west. It goes further to say that "the western quarter gives rise to dryness and dryness gives rise to metal."[7] Dryness in this context refers to a concentration or condensation of essences, a hardening and a receding of moisture from the leaf and stem of plants to the deep interior where it can be safely guarded and preserved.

We see this quality of withdrawal and protection in *xi* 西, the Chinese word for west. The character is an image of a bird coming to roost in the nest as the sun presses down and then sets in the western sky. With this character, we again recognize the connection between the Metal Element and descent, withdrawal and darkness. The association between Metal and the character for west tells us that we are entering a time when the flight of the upper spirits is curtailed. The *shen*, in the form of a bird, descends from the infinite airy heights to settle into the matrix or nest of matter. This gives us a clue to the nature of Metal's spirit and points to a link between the *po*, the setting sun, darkness, matter and the physical body.

The oldest known Chinese glyph for *po* comes from Bronze Script 1700 BCE. It is a picture of a dancing spirit beside a waxing crescent moon with the canopy of Heaven pressing down and protecting them. The character is also sometimes referred to as lunar brightness, which is another way of describing the *po* soul and the yin reflective illumination of this spirit of the underworld.

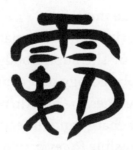

PO - LUNAR BRIGHTNESS

The ancient character tells us that the *po* is related to the hidden, the night and the reflective light of the moon rather than the radiant light of the sun and stars.

The more recent Chinese character for *po* 魄 is formed by placing the radical *ba* 白 white next to the character *gui* 鬼 ghost or spirit:

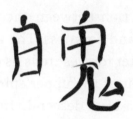

CONTEMPORARY CHARACTER: *PO* SOUL

White is the color of the light of the moon as opposed to the gold of the sun. For the Chinese, it is also the color of death and bones buried beneath the earth. The association with bones emphasizes the *po*'s intrinsic connection to the underworld and the deep structures of the body. But the radical also contains a paradox. The line rising from the top of the graphic for *ba* is sometimes said to represent the light of the rising sun coming up over the eastern horizon. It reminds us that in death, darkness, impasse and decay, new life and resurrection are implicit.

The *po* can be described as the somatic expression of the soul. It is the aspect of the subtle body that organizes the organism, regulates physiology and controls the autonomic nervous system. It manages the breath, peristalsis, sensation, balance, emotional discharge and the capacity for movement. In fact, the *po* is responsible for every part of our being that is indispensable for life.

According to ancient Chinese embryology, the *shen* is the first spirit to arrive at conception—at the moment the sperm actually penetrates the ovum—but as soon as the unformed mass of embryonic cells travels down the fallopian tube to adhere and stick to the wall of the uterus, the energy of the *po* soul constellates. Simultaneous with the fetal linking with the tissue of the mother's body and the first absorption of maternal nutrients, the *po* soul begins its work of organizing anatomical structure and growth. Both the *po* and the fetus are fed by the nutrients and yin essences that pour from the mother's body. As the essences arrive, the *po* moves them and organizes them into form. Then, like the crescent moon that swells with light as it waxes, the mother's belly swells and the baby grows.

Nine months later, when the infant emerges from the womb, takes its first breath and separates from the mother's body, the *po* soul separates from its matrix in the lower cauldron of the body. The breathy *hun* lifts the *po* soul from the Intestines into the Lungs and the life of the individual person begins.

The *po* is responsible for life support and all necessary physiological processes from our birth until our death. From the first breath, the senses—the ears, eyes and Heart—are alive to perception. The hands and feet move. Breathing, appetite and tears, all the basic functions of survival, are already activated. This confirms the idea that during the first month of life, a baby is all *po*, while the *shen*, *hun* and *yi* and even the *zhi* are still developing.

At death, at the last breath, the *po* and *hun* separate. The *hun* follows the *shen* through the Governing Vessel 20 - One Hundred Meetings - *Bai Hui* at the top of the head. The *po* sinks down to the Large Intestine where it rests, adhering to the physical form until the structures of the body begin to decompose and, at last, it returns to the underworld.

The *po* is made up of a consortium of seven part souls, each of whom governs an aspect of our instinctual, animal nature. Each of the seven *po* souls has a vital role to play in the survival and healthy functioning of the body. However, to fulfill their function of sustaining the life of the physical body, these part souls need to be connected to the upper spirits, governed by the directives of the *shen* and the *hun*. If the *shen* are not sufficiently present and rooted in the Heart due to trauma, shock, spirit-level disturbances or congenital weaknesses, the thread of connection between the upper and lower spirits is broken. Then the *po* are vulnerable to the chaotic energies of instinctual drives gone wild. Destructive impulses turn these helpful allies into demonic forces, which express in the form of addictions, self-sabotaging habits and compulsions. Despite their potential for malevolence, however, the *po* souls in all their many forms have a crucial role to play in the mystery of psycho-spiritual transformation.

In the sacred mountain that is the symbol of the self, the *po* resides in the labyrinths and caves that twist and turn deep below the surface of the earth. This dark underworld geography is the symbolic correlate of the lower alchemical cauldron of the body, the Large Intestine, the reproductive organs, the autonomic nervous system and the personal unconscious. In the dark recesses of this underworld, the *po* carry on their sacred tasks of maintaining, protecting and caring for the physical vessel of the soul.

Metal's spirit question: Am I capable of receiving inspiration, letting go and being in the mystery?

Spirit Animal: The White Tiger

The spirit of the Lung has the shape of a White Tiger. Her back is curved around to protect her vulnerable belly. The Lungs hang down like an upside-down bowl or lotus blossom to form a roof to protect the Heart in the upper mansion of the chest. The pale white Lungs hang down as the White Tiger hangs down from her tree and the crescent moon hangs down from the Heavens. Like the *po*, the White Tiger is heavy and stays on the ground. By day, she sleeps. By night, she descends the mountain to hunt in the darkness.

The White Tiger's spirit name is White Splendor. Her given name is Perfection of the Emptiness. Her color is *ba* 白 white, like the essence of the moon.

The White Tiger is very rare. Like Metal, she represents the true yin and is very precious. Like the Lung, the White Tiger is filled with qi that gives her strength and power. But also like the Lung, she must not cling to her fullness. She must be able to let go, breathe out and be empty in order to live. To know fullness as well as emptiness—this is the perfection of the White Tiger.

The White Tiger is a very wild and aggressive animal. She fiercely protects her territory. We find the White Tiger on the warrior's shield as a symbol of protection. "Do not aggress me!" the White Tiger says. So this spirit animal forms a *wei qi*—an outer energetic shield—to protect our bodies and our souls from pathogens and demons.

Leader of all the mountain animals, the wind follows her wherever she goes. The White Tiger is difficult to see but it is important to keep looking for her.

The White Tiger is the protector of the western direction and the harbinger of Autumn. We call on the White Tiger to accompany us when we travel down into the underworld, face our shadow or deal with loss. Placing the image of the White Tiger on a shield over the Heart will protect you from demons and help you see the path of your Tao, even when it is night and the light of the sun is buried below the horizon.

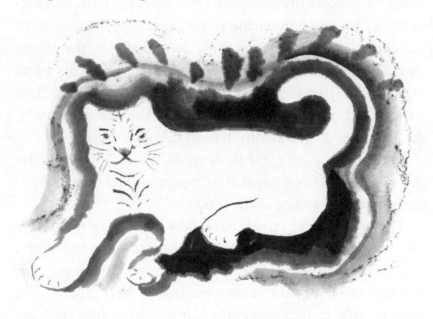

THE WHITE TIGER

Archetype: The Shadow

Modern Western culture encounters the Metal Element and the *po* soul with resistance and denial. The conscious ego experiences this phase of the *sheng* cycle as an assault to its existence, which in many ways it is. The reality of death, the limitations of embodiment and the unruly pull of the instincts remind the ego that it is not always the master of its own house. Consciousness responds by clinging ever more ferociously to the yang and to the illusory permanence of negentropy in the form of youth, power, material accumulations and anything else that temporarily allows it to "beat death." But when we refuse to embrace the ego-defying truths of Metal, the inevitability of loss and the dissolution of the physical body, we also lose our connection to its healing potency. We lose connection to Metal's capacity for transformation and renewal along with our embodied relationship with the Divine.

The Metal Element expresses much that human consciousness rejects and so one of its primary archetypes is the Shadow. The Shadow is an entity universally present in human cultures. C. G. Jung recognized it as a primary archetype of the human collective unconscious. Jung spoke of the integration of the Shadow as "the 'apprentice piece' in the individual's development"[8] and one of the first and most important steps in the individuation process.

The personal Shadow represents the part of us that we reject, repress and deny in order to preserve our conscious identity or "ego ideal." Most often, the Shadow has something to do with our lower spirits, our instinctual or animal nature. Splitting off from the Shadow is the psyche's response to the necessary restrictions and requirements of civilization. It is born of the clash between authentic individual nature and the values and needs of the collective.

But there is also a collective Shadow that constellates when a culture is at odds with the realities of natural and cosmic law. Currently, Western culture has relegated the domain of the lower spirits, particularly the *po* soul, to this shadowy underworld. The collective rejection of body wisdom, the yin and the intimate connection between life and death plays a huge role in both the physical and the psycho-spiritual problems of human beings on the planet at present. Our inability to honor this domain results in physical symptoms such as irritable bowel syndromes, digestive disturbances and obesity and psychological symptoms such as depression, anxiety and addiction.

Even in ancient times, when the individuated ego was still in its infancy and human culture was more closely allied with organic life-and-death processes, the power of Metal was awe-inspiring and difficult to fathom. In Taoist mythology, Metal became associated with the *gui*, the ghosts or wandering disembodied souls of the shadow lands. Initially, there was no evil connotation to this term. Rather than being viewed as dangerous demons, *gui* were regarded as expressions of Divine energy, natural forces, earthly spirits that were the counter-pole to the *shen*. At this early time, the *gui* could be viewed as closely allied with the Greek idea of a *daemon*, a spirit guide or Divine internal life force that shapes the bodily form but also inspires and calls forth the soul into life.

After the introduction of Buddhism into China and as world culture moved toward increased rejection of the yin, the notion of the *gui* shifted. The character changed to its more modern form 鬼, a big head and a small body, and was described as a monster with a tail, a starving ghost that could never be satisfied. The *gui* were relegated to the dangerous misty swamplands and deserted night shadows of graveyards. Rather than being viewed as an aspect of the body soul and an important part of the dance of life, they were increasingly connected with evil yin possession states and the malcontented spirits of the dead.

The *gui* can be viewed as manifestations of the psychic energy of the unconscious and body. As such, their impulses and agendas are often at odds with the goals of our conscious mind. But when we attempt to project, deny or annihilate the disorienting and seemingly antagonistic impulses that arise from our lower spirit, we lose touch with our *daemon*, our inspiring life force, as well as the enlivening potency of the opposites that is the essence of alchemical transformation.

As we become conscious of our own Shadow, no matter how

difficult, alien or disturbing it may be, we discover more about ourselves and our authentic nature and come closer to our Tao, recognizing and relating to this part of becoming a whole and healthy human being. It can help us to access our own authenticity, potency and dimensionality and the exuberance and initiative often lacking in our upper ego consciousness.

Next time you find yourself upset, irritated or resentful of another person, take a step back and ask yourself if there is something about this person that might remind you of a part of yourself you have rejected. This is what I call "eating your own Shadow." It may not taste good but it will ultimately nourish your soul. As you "take back" the projection of your Shadow and own it as a part of you, get curious about what it wants and needs. Reflect on what you can do to honor but not be taken over by it. This is the beginning of transforming a destabilizing demon into a daemon, an inspiring and helpful friend.

Alchemy: Transforming Grief into Presence

As I walk alone through the late November twilight, I notice that the air is filled with emptiness. October's multicolored patchwork of leaves is now a straggle of torn gold rattling on bare black branches. The veil between the worlds of life and death has grown thin.

Sometimes I go to sit on a stone and watch the water. This stone, where my mother also sat in summer for so many years, is now cold. One night, I saw my mother spread the wings of her white nightgown and lift into the Heavens. I miss her every day, and this missing reminds me of clouds, of something precious that is slipping through my fingers like a fine silk thread.

One day, I walked down to the shore and saw that the land

had been broken open. A hole had been dug and a foundation poured. Someone had put up a sign that said the waters were dead and the cove polluted. I did not want to go back, but I have returned to watch the tide and the small brown ducks who like to winter over here.

Metal requires that we not turn back from the darkness. It invites us to breathe deep into loss and not avert our gaze from the tragedy of our own story, our own time. Metal tells me that if I turn away from what I cannot bear, my life will be lost to me.

Often, the sadness feels too painful. Words scatter in the winds of the underworld and all I want to do is close my eyes and sleep. But, taking my time, breathing into my grief, saying yes instead of no to the restriction and the loss, something opens in my Heart.

In this way, I can stay present in my circumstances. In this way, I can dare to leap into a night without dreams, without bottom and without end. I can wait. I can listen. And when I hear the White Tiger in the darkness, I can follow where it leads me.

Metal Spirit Points

Lung 1 - Middle Palace - *Zhong Fu*
中府

In late day light,
birch groves ignite and wordless,
I watch as night falls.

This point is like a day in mid-autumn when distilled sunlight pours through the tree branches, turning the burnished leaves into the stained-glass windows of a celestial palace. The mansion of the chest spontaneously expands as the breath rushes in to catch this last glimmer of Fire—the final turning point—before the descent into the cold grays and blues of Winter.

Fu or palace points have the special capacity to govern over their meridian. Lung 1 - Middle Palace - *Zhong Fu* 中府 is the first point on the Lung meridian. It opens us to the entire passage of the Metal Element, from inhalation to exhalation, from the fierce White Tiger of the *wei qi*—the yang protective energy layer of immunity that lies just above the skin—to the tender yin sensitivity of the curling air passages of the nose and Lungs. From the first lusty desirous howl of life to the gossamer thread of the last breath, this point enlivens and regulates the movement of the qi through the Lung meridian.

Middle Palace - *Zhong Fu* is the palace in the middle, between inhalation and exhalation, between Heaven and Earth. When we touch Middle Palace - *Zhong Fu*, we open a conduit between the Heavenly and Earthly aspects of the self. As the chest expands and the breath of Heaven fills our Lungs, we feel the mystery of spirit infuse our corporeal being. The point, which is the anatomical counterpoint to Bladder 42 (or 37) - Door of Corporeal Soul - *Po Hu*,[9] supports the corporeal soul in restoring the rhythmic harmony of Heaven and Earth, spirit and matter, yang and yin in the various autonomic processes of the body.

Zhong 中 is a square with a line down the middle. It is said to be a picture of an arrow hitting the center of a target. The character expresses in graphic form the energy of righteous Metal—the capacity to stay centered in the preciousness of the moment, to be exactly present where I am right here, right now—while acknowledging and appreciating the ephemeral nature of time, which is always passing.

Fu 府 is a picture of a hand turning something over—a payment, handshake of agreement or commitment—taking place under the cover of 广 a roof that functions to protect the transaction. So at the spiritual center of this point, under the protection of the latticework of bones that make up our rib cage, an agreement is being made that with each breath, we commit anew to our Tao and to the preciousness of our life.

This point is the entry point of the Lung meridian. When needled or activated after Liver 14 - Gate of Hope - *Qi Men*, the exit point of the Liver, it reinvigorates hope, inspiration and vision. Opening Gate of Hope - *Qi Men* followed by Middle Palace - *Zhong Fu* allows us to receive the potency of sky qi and the energies of Heaven so that we can bear the limitations and losses of life and still remain present to the sacred preciousness of each moment.

Consider this point as an ally when there is coughing, breathing difficulties, anxious feelings in the chest, an inability to surrender to grief and tears and resistance to new possibilities, inner preciousness and inspiration.

Suggested Flower Essence: Yerba Santa

Yerba santa means "holy herb" and the essence made from the flowers of this plant helps us to rediscover the sacredness of our life. When grief has been buried in the Heart, yerba santa allows us to release it. In particular, this flower essence opens up the mansion of the chest. It is particularly useful when grief has become rock hard through constraint and tears are crystallized. The breathing becomes constricted and life loses its vibrancy. Yerba santa reverses this process by gradually softening our resistance to loss, gently opening the chest and allowing us to renew our connection to life and the self.

Also consider adding five rice grain moxa lit directly on this point in order to further reignite the warmth, suppleness and luminosity of the Metal Element. The light and warmth of the moxa illuminate Middle Palace - *Zhong Fu* so that we can perceive and feel the awesome mystery of the spirit in the midst of our material existence. By warming and softening the muscles of the chest wall, moxa on this point supports the release of held breath and allows for the flow of necessary tears. Following moxa with the penetration of a slender needle touches the soul like a ray of sunlight piercing the shadows of a birch grove in the late autumn twilight.

Lung 2 - Cloud Gate - *Yun Men*

雲門

Parting now, the clouds
reveal their luminous wings. Smoke-like,
ghosts spiral into light.

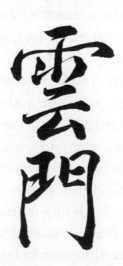

Last weeks of autumn. The multicolored patchwork of early autumn is now a straggling of gold leaves rattling on bare black branches. The veil between the worlds grows thin and we feel the nights come closer. Nature invites us to slow down, to look within and to reflect on the essence of who we truly are.

At times when we cannot see beyond the mists, at times of uncertainty, loss and letting go, this point opens our Lungs and allows us to breathe more freely. On a spirit level, it opens a passageway in the clouds so that our souls can see what we truly need.

The character *yun* 雲, meaning cloud, is closely related to the ancient character meaning to say or speech. One hidden power of Lung 2 - Cloud Gate - *Yun Men* 雲門 is its capacity to open the gate of the throat so that we can speak from our truth, so that we can give voice to our authentic nature. Speaking in this way brings clarity, light and inspiration back to our world. Consider this point when there is not enough talking or too much talking, when there is no trust in silence.

This point opens a small passageway in the mist so that we can accept the wisdom of loss and remember the preciousness of darkness. After loss, depression, oppression and death, Cloud Gate - *Yun Men* clears a way for the soul to move on, to prepare for the next stage of the journey of embodied life. It allows us to rest in the spaciousness of grief and to rediscover our faith in emptiness.

Consider this point when a person has forgotten his or her own preciousness or the preciousness of others, and when the world has forgotten the preciousness of life itself, the preciousness of each passing moment. Other indications include mourning that has persisted beyond its appropriate course of time, an unwillingness to let go and trust the next breath and a sense that the soul is shrouded in depression or confusion. I have also found this point effective when there is a cloudy or muffled quality to the Lung pulse, especially when there is repressed grief or emerging trauma memories.

When we dip the needle into this point, the spirit relaxes back into the spaciousness of time and we rediscover our faith in surrender. The breath returns, bringing life and vitality back to the body. Through the action of Cloud Gate - *Yun Men*, the *po* soul's tendency toward turbidity, stuckness and tenacious gripping is lightened, lifted and liberated. We remember that the world is wide and the unexpected may at times be miraculous. The clouds part and the gates of inspiration open to reveal a sunlit sky, infinite in its grace.

Suggested Essential Oil: Ravensara

This oil clears oppression and also protects strongly against toxic influences at a physical and a psycho-spiritual level. It supports the resilience of the immune system. It opens the Lungs to the breath and the soul to new possibilities. Ravensara is enlivening and invigorating. It is useful for allergies and bronchitis on a physical level but also for when a person can't see through the film of their own phlegm, the accumulation of their life thoughts and experiences. Needling Cloud Gate - *Yun Men* clears away the clouds that block us from our Tao. Moxa to this point warms our spirit. And Ravensara applied here will protect us from toxic influences and help release the ghosts of the past to allow us to move forward into the future.

Lung 3 - Palace of Heaven - *Tian Fu*
天府

In this dark mansion,
blossoms of breath instead of flowers.
Gassho! I lift my head towards Heaven.

Lung 3 - Palace of Heaven - *Tian Fu* 天府 brings the energy of early autumn when the softly ripening light of Earth season turns bright and crisp. You look up to the clear cerulean blue of the October sky and feel spirits everywhere.

We open this Window-to-the-Sky point in order to catch a glimpse of the other side of grief. When this point is ready to be needled, it means that the dues have been paid. The time of mourning is coming to an end. It is the right moment to let go of the ones we have loved who have passed and open our eyes again to life as it is.

In this mansion, the Divine is revealed as a space of meeting, the place where I open my palm to another, to give and to receive. Palace of Heaven - *Tian Fu* lets the light of the breath illuminate the upper mansion of the chest and allows us to discover our true treasure. The payment to be made is not in coins but in the release, in the opening of the empty palm.

Consider this point when it is time to wash the windows of the soul, after the death of someone or some part of the self. It supports us in seeing our life in a new way, recognizing the majesty of our being. This is a point that has the power to calm the *po* soul and modulate the weeping, disorientation and lassitude of grief. In ancient folklore and traditional medicine, it is recognized as a point that can clear away ghosts and demons. We can reframe this in modern psychological terms as a capacity to support recovery from shock and trauma, especially when a person is "haunted" by memory, is overwhelmed by emotion or is in a state of disassociation from their own being.

Suggested Essential Oil: Frankincense

Frankincense helps us to overcome stress and despair and to rediscover a sense of spiritual connection. It allows us to experience the sacredness of loss and to open ourselves to the support of energies that come from beyond our own limited conscious awareness. It supports the healing of old scars and promotes a sense of protection from negative influences. Consider frankincense when a person needs to find acceptance, surrender and inspiration.

Lung 8 - Meridian Gutter - *Jing Qu*
經渠

As I clear leaves from the roof drain,
a last cricket laughs.
Here comes another gust of wind!

Lung 8 - Meridian Gutter - *Jing Qu* 經渠 is like a rainy day with leaves falling in clusters from the trees, collecting in piles of brown, crimson and gold in damp corners of the garden.

This point is not often used in modern acupuncture practice, but in my early studies, my teacher, J. R. Worsley, emphasized its value. We turn to this point in the autumn, a season that all traditional healing and spiritual systems recognize as a time of clearing and letting go. As the leaves fall from the trees, we are called to shed parts of ourselves we no longer need. And as the energies of the yin and of entropy are on the rise, life slows down, the forces of initiatory movement decline and things tend to accumulate. Falling leaves gather in rag-tag piles and come to rest in low places like gutters and streams and our own energies may tend to stagnate. Old attitudes, emotions and thoughts, like accumulated toxins, resist moving on.

This is the point to call on when the organism's dispersal capacities are challenged. On a physical level, this point can be used to clear phlegm and to relieve coughing and asthma. On a psycho-spiritual level, it is useful when we need to clear out "old stuff," to dredge our psychological drains of "leaves," of what is "left over," so that the waters of our life can flow. The ancient indication of this point as a distal point for the relief of pain of the sole of the foot can be translated on the psycho-spiritual level as an ability to support us in "walking," in moving forward in our life.

This point invites us to ask: what has accumulated that is now getting in my way? In autumn, what do I need to clear away in order to prepare for the rains and snows of winter?

Lung 9 - Supreme Abyss - *Tai Yuan*

太淵

> *Harvest moon long gone,*
> *I stand alone on the bridge.*
> *Below me, black water rises.*

Cold, wet fog envelops the trees and the world heads downward toward the yin. It is a day of letting go: at its worst, depression; at its best, a surrender to transformation. Cricket and frog songs are gone. Now, only the last few sparrows peck hungrily at seeds on the bare branches.

We open Lung 9 - Supreme Abyss - *Tai Yuan* 太淵 when a person's grief has become too heavy for them to bear. Something larger is needed to help hold the tears. The abyss is very deep. It extends down into the far interiority of the chest. This point brings a breath of fresh air to the Lungs and Heart. It allows for the receiving of blood, forgotten stories that need to be told. This point reminds us that in the deepest, most abysmal place, we discover hidden starlight.

The "greatness" of this point reminds us that the depths are connected to the Heavens. The breath lifts the *po* soul up from its state of yin isolation and interiority into a lively connection with the sensory world.

Suggested Essential Oil: Atlas Cedar

The Atlas cedar tree is native to the Atlas mountains of North Africa. It is long-lived and typically reaches heights of 150 feet or more. The inner heart of this tree is a warm mahogany red, the color of the alchemical metal, cinnabar. For millennia, the wood of cedar trees has been recognized for its capacity to repel insects and resist decay. It has been used as a sacred incense and as a building material for temples, tombs and ocean-going vessels.

Applied to the Supreme Abyss - *Tai Yuan*, the oil of the Atlas cedar helps to transform phlegm on a physical and a psychological level. In this way, it brings vitality and clarity to the body, mind and soul. It offers strength and steadfastness in times of crisis. It strengthens spiritual certainty and restores the connection between individual and cosmic will. When there is resistance to letting go and moving forward, this oil helps eliminate fear, banish guilt and endow us with trust in the unknown and the courage to risk taking action for ourselves when appropriate.

The cinnabar color of the Atlas cedar heartwood accentuates the relationship of its oil to alchemy and to the Heart. By connecting the Lungs with the Heart, the oil of the resilient, tall and upright tree helps to transform our resistance to change and fear of death into an acceptance of and receptivity to mystery.

Lung 10 - Fish Region - *Yu Ji*
魚祭

*Goldfish blaze shadows
in a black pond. Flickering fire.
Ignites the darkness.*

There are days in late autumn when a kind of Fire leaps upward from the waning energies of the yang. We see it in the brilliance of the sunset, the last rich crimson of the maple leaves and the determined vitality in the air. And yet the ephemeral nature of this Fire is palpable, the sunsets swallowed by the swiftly approaching night and the bright color of the leaves fading with the twilight.

I consider Lung 10 - Fish Region - *Yu Ji* 魚祭 as a door to the region of the *po*, the lower soul. The point allows us to touch the light of spirit that glows from the matrix of matter. As the Fire in the Metal point, I turn to Fish Region - *Yu Ji* when the Metal has lost its warmth and luster.

I called on the medicine of this point for a woman whose mother has died six months earlier. She arrived for her session wondering why she was feeling foggy and tired. Although she claimed that everything was "really fine," I could see that she was not.

"What is wrong with me?" she asks.

"Your mother just died, less than a year ago," I say.

She looks at me, a bit shocked and nods her head, yes. As she realizes that she is still mourning, she begins to cry. Light returns to her eyes and her breathing deepens.

I needle Fish Region - *Yu Ji* with a small, slender needle to support this kind of surrendering to grief, this settling into self-awareness. Through the recognition and acceptance of the suffering and loss that is an inevitable part of embodied life, we discover a deeper connection to the self and to the Divine. Used in this way, the point does not erase grief but rather enhances grief's capacity to open us to the preciousness of life by softening, warming and brightening the Metal Element. It connects the Lungs and the Heart and supports Metal's capacity for receptivity, its ability to receive and cherish and to surrender and let go.

Suggested Treatment Strategy: Rice Grain Moxa and Essential Oil

Fish Region - *Yu Ji* is an exquisitely tender, sensitive point that responds rapidly to even very light needling. I go in with clear intention, care and deep respect for the point's depth and power. Sometimes, even one rice grain moxa is enough, sometimes three, rarely, if ever, more. Moxa on this point brings the spirit back to life after loss. It sends a current of warming Fire through the upper mansion of the chest, softening the armoring of the intercostal muscles and allowing the Heart and the Lungs to open to the spaciousness and transformational potential of grief.

Large Intestine 5 - Yang Stream - *Yang Xi*
陽溪

Grasping the last green
carrot top, I pull. From cold earth:
comes sunshine.

A crisp wind in the trees challenges the old order, winnows out what is not strong enough to withstand the winter. Today, there is a pale sun with a determined warmth and brightness. In the midst of the cooling season, there is still an underground Fire.

Large Intestine 5 - Yang Stream - *Yang Xi* 陽溪 brings light, warmth and vitality. It counterbalances Metal's innate tendency to become cold, rigid and still when divorced from Fire. It restores the spirit of the yang even as the cosmic Fire dwindles.

The first time I experienced this point was in early November. I was still a student, living in Baltimore. I was fighting a cold as the weather shifted from the balmy warmth of mid-Atlantic late summer to the cold, damp chill of the city's version of autumn. I was feeling tired, lonely and cut off from my own enthusiasm and joy. Moxa and needling on this point produced an immediate shift in the area of my Heart and Lungs. A flow of warmth and wellbeing traveled up my arms to my chest and then through my whole being. I felt strong and safe, as if I had donned a bright armor of protection. I could face the chill wind with a sense of strength and endurance.

I turn to this point when I want to restore warmth and flow to the Metal Element. I consider it when a person is stuck in a rigid pattern of resistance to change, locked in grief or doubtful of their ability to receive the inspiration of spirit. A current of warming water flows through the soul so that once again, light can shine from the stream bed of being.

Looking to the hidden message of the point name, we note that the character *xi* 洗 stream also means to shower, wash or bathe and, in rare instances, is also used to mean baptize. From this, we can understand that Yang Stream - *Yang Xi* is a point that washes us with warm water, showers away accumulated dirt and debris and offers a renewal of spirit, a baptism of light and warmth as we enter the darker, colder time of the year.

Suggested Essential Oil: Cinnamon Leaf

Cinnamon leaf is a warming, spicy oil that invigorates the blood, revives the senses and activates our internal resources so that we can face the challenges of the environment more effectively. It provides a feeling of protection as we move out into the world. In addition, by invigorating the blood and warming the interior, it allows us to communicate more easily with our inner selves, to know what we truly need in order to survive and flourish.

This is a perfect oil to turn to when the Fire Element is not bringing its gifts or warmth and illumination to the Metal, when Metal has grown brittle and cold and we want to help a person restore a connection to their own Heart. Through this connection to self, we come back to a sense of our own unique preciousness along with our capacity for relatedness to others.

Large Intestine 6 - Veering Passage - *Pian Li*
偏歷

Racket of pine,
ruckus of rose hip, black-capped
chickadees prepare for snow.

The seasons do not move from one to the next in a smoothly flowing pattern. Rather, the cosmic energies come together like the tides of rivers, weather streams creating shocks, eddies and waves as the new patterns take over the old. As the season turns from autumn to winter, there are days that feel jagged and a bit disturbing. We do not know if it is going to snow or simply go on with icy rain. In the garden, animals and birds pick up the pace of their gathering and feeding. They run and flit in and out between the trees, not in the relaxed, leisurely graceful lines of summer, but with a kind of erratic frenzy that can seem purposeless but is, in fact, precise in its intent to survive.

Large Intestine 6 - Veering Passage - *Pian Li* 偏歷 is the *luo*-connecting point on the Large Intestine meridian. It is related to the *luo* point, Lung 7 - Broken Sequence - *Lie Que* 列缺. Both points are located slightly off the expected line of the meridian in surprisingly sensitive hollows on the arm. This "veering" off the line tells us something about the nature and wisdom of this point.

Touching this point affirms our knowing that the Way is not always a straight path. And yet, as this point opens the flow of qi down the arm, into the index finger and up into the orifices of the head, it empowers our ability to point our way forward, to see where we need to go despite the twists and turns of the journey. We turn to this point at the later stage of the grieving process, as we begin to truly release the soul of the being we have lost or the familiar but outmoded behavior patterns of our past.

Suggested Essential Oil: Clary Sage

This oil allows us to see clearly and, like the owl, to see what we need when we are traveling in the dark. Clary sage relaxes tension, benefits the Lungs and respiratory system and brings a rush of mental–emotional uplift. I like to use this oil on Veering Passage - *Pian Li* to enliven sensory awareness and promote acuity of perception, especially in regard to what we need in order to survive. It helps us to trust that we can see clearly despite the inevitable twists and turns of life's path.

Large Intestine 11 - Pool at the Crook - *Qu Chi*
曲池

Quarry where I swam
now cold and quiet. Dragonflies turned
to drifting leaves.

One of Ma Danyang's Twelve Heavenly Star Points and Sun Simiao's Thirteen Ghost Points, we know that Large Intestine 11 - Pool at the Crook - *Qu Chi* 曲池 has had special significance to practitioners over the centuries. As a Heavenly Star Point, it is used to clear Fire that transmits to the Heart and spirit and is particularly indicated for agitation, depression and oppression of the chest. As a Ghost Point, it is used to calm manic states and settle the soul. As the Earth in the Metal point, it actively clears and transforms any last remnants of Late Summer and disperses phlegm, heat and wind.

The point name includes the character *chi* 池 pool. The character is made up of two parts, the abbreviated radical for water alongside the phonetic that derives from a stylized picture of a woman's genitals, also sometimes described as a "she-snake." The inclusion of this deeply yin element in the point name tells us something about the potency and mystery of this point, its capacity to move, dredge and transform. It also reminds us that this point can function as a doorway to deep places in the soul and psyche and can be used to help dislodge ghosts and soften outmoded emotional holding patterns.

On a physical level, it is effective for treating acute sore throat, laryngitis and toothache and for clearing heat and fever. On a spirit level, I turn to this point when grief has been buried and has turned to a kind of hidden heat, almost impossible to touch. Needling this point is the equivalent of coming across an unexpected source of water that can cool, clear and encourage the life force to renew. It is a point of fundamental release of both acute and chronic holding patterns.

Like any hidden pond or pool that one finds when walking along a crooked path in a forest, this point is a gathering place for spirits and ghosts. We come here to help the *po* soul let go of what it no longer needs to carry. In this way, we begin to release grief, trauma and outmoded holding patterns on a cellular level.

Pool at the Crook - *Qu Chi* opens us to our depths and allows the life force to flow. It brings Metal's wisdom of the deep yin surrender. It clears accumulations on every level and brings release and calm receptivity to the soul.

Suggested Essential Oil: Cypress

Cypress clears heat from the blood and vigorously enlivens and regulates blood flow. It is an anti-spasmodic, cool and astringing. On a physical level, it helps heal the throat, calms a spastic colon and eases menstrual cramps. It transforms damp and clears the mind.

On a psycho-spiritual level, the cypress tree has long been associated with the healing of grief. Its unique upright oval form with an elongated tip pointing toward the sky instills a feeling of hope in the face of death and loss. The cypress tree has been used as a symbol of mourning in both Eastern and Western cultures for thousands of years. The Japanese revered it as one of the five sacred trees. In ancient Greece, it was planted at sites that were considered doorways to the underworld. Native tribes of the American Southwest regarded this tree with reverence, and all over the world, from New England to Italy to Israel to the Middle East to China, we find cypress trees planted beside graves and at the entry to cemeteries.

At the same time, because of its hardiness and longevity, cypress has been associated with rejuvenation and long life. As a blood-moving tonic, it helps us to be more at ease with emotion and to clear trauma. This oil can help us be more comfortable with our grief, to surrender to the healing gift of our tears and to realign ourselves with life in the face of destabilizing experiences of loss and change.

Large Intestine 18 - Support and Rush Out - *Fu Tu*

扶突

V of geese beneath
Hunter's Moon.
I wake to salute their passing.

A day in autumn when the energies of the world are on the move. Squirrels run wildly back and forth, digging holes to store acorns and nuts for the winter. The wind rushes through the trees and flocks of birds interrupt the vastness of the sky. Fox skulk in the field and deer graze hungrily on the last fallen apples. There is a wildness, a vitality that comes with finally letting go and trusting the process of transformation that is underway in the world.

Large Intestine 18 - Support and Rush Out - *Fu Tu* 扶突 is the window of the sky of the Large Intestine meridian. We consider opening the windows when it is time for a new outlook. As these points are all located in the area between the upper chest and head, they are also important when a person needs to make some new connections between their mind and body, thoughts and actions. In the words of physician Zhou Zhi-Cong in his commentary to the *Yellow Emperor's Classics*, these points are "the great windows of a high pavilion by virtue of which qi moves."[10]

The commonly accepted indications for this point are coughing, wheezing, loss of voice, physical difficulty with swallowing and chronic disorders of the vocal cords. But when we look deeper to the point's spiritual nature, we discover that it has a much greater purpose. When I clear and release the throat, I am preparing to open my entire being to the world. I am preparing to allow my self to sound out. And yet, when Support and Rush Out - *Fu Tu* is called for, something holds back in the face of the release. The voice does not come easily. You have a sense that the animal is stuck in its hole—needing to move, to sound, to speak, to come out from hiding.

When I needle this point, I am supporting my own and my patient's capacity to express creativity and aliveness even in the face of limitations and the inevitable challenges of Winter. The name of this point reminds us that in order to truly trust and open the voice of self out into the world, we need to feel the deep support of the body and the Earth below us, but also the support of another, a listener—in this case, the hand of the practitioner who holds the needle.

The radical *fu* 扶, with its graphic of the supporting hand that helps, relieves and straightens, makes the importance of relationship abundantly clear when we approach this point. As it is located on the neck, between the two heads of the sternocleidomastoid muscle, even touching this point with the fingers creates a feeling of tremendous vulnerability. Always ask before approaching and remember the power of this point when opening it.

Suggested Flower Essence: Trumpet Vine

Trumpet vine is a perennial climbing vine with a vibrant abundance of bright orange, trumpet-shaped flowers that bloom in mid-summer. The flower essence made from the blossoms of this plant promotes a sense of vitality and presence, a willingness to open our throat and trust the unimpeded expression of the voice of the self.

Large Intestine 20 - Welcome Fragrance - *Ying Xiang*

迎香

After the storm, a downed pine,
a warming wind and a moon
the color of roses.

By the last weeks of November, the scent of the natural world has already taken on the transparency of winter. A series of bitterly cold nights has dispersed the rich aroma of evergreen, mudflats, mushrooms, humus and moss, leaving a clear, ice-water flavor to the air. But after a torrential rainstorm and a rising, warm west wind, I go out for a walk and discover that the woods are once again infused with the smell of sap and decay, of green essences and fur and the dreaming of growth. It is as if the season is offering me a parting gift, a token of affection and an assurance that, after winter's deep freeze, life's potency will return from the underworld, bringing movement, vitality, color and flavor back along with it. I raise my head and sniff the wind like a dog. I inhale deeply. This will keep me for a while.

Large Intestine 20 - Welcome Fragrance - *Ying Xiang* 迎香 is a point that is often used to clear nasal congestion, rhinitis, runny nose, loss of smell and taste. It is so effective, at times with almost shocking immediacy, that it is easy to forget its psycho-spiritual effects, its capacity to clear the mind and reinvigorate the senses.

To understand the deeper psychological relevance of this point, we turn to the Chinese character *zi* 自 self, which etymologically is described as a picture of a nose! It turns out that one pointed to one's nose to say, "I am," and to indicate the miraculous life-giving infusion of breath and spirit that was recognized as the animating force of the self in ancient China. Through the action of this point, I come back to my self and remember the sweet fragrance of the spirit world that infuses the world of matter.

Suggested Essential Oil: Scots Pine

Scots pine is a warming, tonifying oil that has a particular affinity to the Lungs and the Metal Element. The tall, gracious pine, reaching up to the airy spaciousness of the sky, has an affinity for the Lungs, the Metal Element and the *po*.

Pine needles have a tremendous potential to oxygenate. On a physical level, pine is an effective remedy for wheezing and shallow breathing. It opens the chest and allows the soul to breathe and take in the life forces of the sky. It opens the airways and invigorates the breath. It is useful for pulmonary complaints and for clearing phlegm from the Lungs. Apply this oil to Lung points when there is exhaustion, wheezing, respiratory congestion and Lung qi deficiency.

On a psycho-emotional level, it disperses melancholy and grief and helps us to reconnect to our deep instinctual energies and zest for life. It opens the mansion of the chest. Pine enlivens the *po*—our animal soul—allowing us to rediscover our own natural rhythms. It brings calm, restores trust in the cycles of life and allows us to surrender to processes of change.

Bladder 42 (or 37) - Door of the Corporeal Soul - *Po Hu*

魄戶

Bare branches catch stars
in their tattered nets. One twig snaps...
and springs the trap.

A day at the mid-point of autumn, celebrated as the Day of the Dead, Halloween. This is a day of scudding clouds and wind, leaves already fallen and beginning to rot in clumps in the unraked grass. The veil between the worlds is thin. Spirits rise in spirals from the cooling ground and rush in between the trees. It is a day of dying, letting go. With a deep release of the breath, in the spaciousness of loss, we find a feather touch of longing, a preciousness of presence. No more running. We rest for a moment. We breathe. Here. Now.

The *po* soul is the animating spirit of the body. In Taoist mythology, it is regarded as a messenger who has the ability to travel between the middle realm of Earth and the lower realms of the underworld, the domain of *Xi Wang Mu*, the Queen Mother of the West. The *po* brings the messages of the Dark Goddess back to us in the form of deep body knowing, muscular and neurological responses and the acceptance of loss as a prerequisite of change. At times of crisis, challenge and transition, the *po* supports our capacity to hold steady, to stay "in our bodies" and to accept that larger wisdom lies beyond the limits of our own consciousness.

Bladder 42 (or 37) - Door of the Corporeal Soul - *Po Hu* 魄戶 opens and closes to allow for the soul's need to come and go between worlds. As long as this movement remains fluid, the organism will remain in balance. However, at times, due to shock, loss, physical pain or environmental challenge to the nervous system, the *po* descends to the lower world and does not return in a timely way. Then we see symptoms of disassociation, fatigue, a lack of connection to the world, depression, despair and an inability to grieve, cry or care for the physical body. There may also be psychosomatic symptoms including chest tightness, shallow breathing, skin sensitivity and disorientation.

When the spirit of Metal is weak, when there is no luster to a person's being, no sense of the preciousness of life and no vital connection to the life force, then opening the Door of the Corporeal Soul - *Po Hu* and inviting the *po* to return to the body may be a way to initiate a process of healing.

Suggested Treatment Strategy:
Rice Grain Moxa with Frankincense

I like to use five to seven rice grain moxa on this point to "lift" the *po* back up into the Lungs when a person is dispirited or dejected. I consider using moxa on this point when I have the sense that the *po* has abandoned its lively relationship with the *hun* and the body has lost its delight and shine. After a shock, for emotional vacuity, I use moxa on *Po Hu*, the Door of the Corporeal Soul, to open the wings of the spirit and restore a person's capacity to be inspired.

I follow the moxa on Door of the Corporeal Soul - *Po Hu* with a drop of frankincense essential oil. Frankincense is a small tree that grows in the Middle East and North Africa. The oil is made from resin that is collected from incisions made in the bark of the tree. These incisions leave scars on the trunk as the tree heals, which is related to the use of frankincense as a healer of wounds and scars, whether at the physical, psychological or spiritual level.

Recognized for millennia for its healing properties and unique aroma, the rising smoke of the resin of *Boswellia* or frankincense was an important part of religious ceremonies in Ancient Egypt, Persia, Israel, Greece and Rome. The rising smoke was viewed as a way to carry earthly prayers upward to the Heavens and is said to be one of the gifts of the Magi to the infant Jesus. The burning, richly aromatic resin is still used today in religious rituals around the world.

The oil has a strong effect on the nervous system and helps to alleviate the effects of stress and trauma. It smooths and harmonizes qi and calms the nerves but also has a powerful effect on the Lungs, deepening the breath, relieving tightness in the chest and alleviating the symptoms of sinusitis and laryngitis.

The oil is also known to have profound psychological and spiritual effects. It allows us to experience the sacredness of loss and to open ourselves to the protection and support of energies that come from beyond our own limited conscious awareness. Following moxa on Door of the Corporeal Soul - *Po Hu* with a drop of frankincense essential oil enhances the action of the moxa and further strengthens the relationship between the *po* soul and the *hun*. As the yin *po* is lifted back into connection with the breathy yang *hun*, it is liberated from the grip of gravity and released from its tendency to constriction, addiction and despair. In this way, the weight of matter and the body is lightened and we remember the wings of the soul that are always at our backs.

Conclusion:
Scattering Stardust

Each point is a poem made up of flesh, muscle, tendon, nerve, word, image, soul, emptiness and a bit of starlight. Like a haiku, each point comes to life again and again, a singular event, a moment in time, an awakening to beauty, a unique new possibility. When we approach the points in this way, each practitioner has the opportunity to become an artisan of the life force, a mender of broken wholeness, as well as a clinician and healer. In this way, each treatment becomes a poem for the soul. With each insertion of the needle, a new thread of meaning is woven through the life world, and Heaven and Earth draw closer.

In a brief line taken from one of his poems, the poet Jalal ad-Din Muhammad Rumi wrote, "Inside the needle's eye, a turning night of stars."[1] This line reminds me of the infinite space that we approach through the minute aperture of the point. Sliding through the needle's eye, we enter a different dimension where a turning night of stars, suns, moons, dreams and mysteries opens us to the domain of the spirits.

But the presence of the spirits is not a given. In the realm of embodiment, the spirits only come when we call them, invite them, care about them deeply and open our eyes in such a way that we can perceive their elusive light. They land like birds, bats, moths, butterflies, fragments of meteors, snowflakes, angel wings, moonbeams or a perfectly poised kigo. Then they rest, light as feathers, tiny luminous flames, on the altar of our bodies, on the altar of matter. Through our rituals, our songs, our poetry, our touch, our prayers, our ululations in praise of the natural world, we invite these ephemeral beings to gift us with their light and their messages. Once we are able to see in this way, to hear in this way, it is our task to do whatever we can to root the light of the *shen* in the matrix of matter and the body: as story, as insight, as tear, as dream, as act of daring, benevolence, passion, creativity or faith.

In his book *Existence*, author, poet and translator David Hinton writes:

> The generative life-supporting reality of earth requires the infusion of energies from heaven, energies that evolve through annual patterns creating the seasons: sunlight, rain, snow, air. Indeed, as we now know, earth is made of heaven's scattering of stardust, and will again become heaven when our sun explodes into a nebula that engulfs earth, turning it into stardust. We dwell in our everyday lives at the origin place where this vital intermingling of heaven and earth takes place, at the center of a dynamic cocoon of cosmic energy, an all-encompassing generative present, but we are rarely aware of this wondrous fact.[2]

It is our responsibility, should we feel called to embrace it, as healers at this time of crisis, opportunity and transformation on the planet, to remain in awareness of the wonder. It is our mandate, should we feel brave enough to fulfill it, to take up the task of the shamans, alchemists and healer priests of old who gathered up the luminescence of the night sky and spun it into twirling capes and silver wings. In honor of the craft of the ancient medicine ways, we don our capes and spread our wings. We spin up into the galaxies and down to the depths of the sea, in search of the wisdom, power and sight we need in order to heal and restore holiness to our broken world.

I will admit that my belief in the spirit that resides at the heart of the points and my love and respect for the ancient Japanese haiku poets is, in part, a romantic longing for a different time when magicians danced patterns up star stairs to the clouds, when shamans rode the spring winds on the backs of dragons and the natural world was more intact, more woven with Heaven in and through the texture of our days and nights.

But the truth is that many of the greatest Chinese and Japanese poets, artists, spiritual teachers and healers did not live in ease during times of peace and harmony. More often, they lived during times of chaos and crisis, cultural breakdown, war, economic uncertainty and tyranny. In *Existence*, David Hinton speaks of the landscape artists, Chan poets and Taoist sages who lived in the aftermath of the barbarian takeover that brought destruction and an end to the Ming Dynasty. As acts of resistance to the barbarian rule, these sages, artists and healers took long journeys and deepened their art as a spiritual practice. As Hinton explains, "Artist-intellectuals found their spiritual home in mountains, thought of mountains as their teachers...they lived as much as possible in cultivated reclusion among mountain, wandered mountains...dreamed mountains and built their creative lives around them."[3]

As I reflect on the uncertainty of our time and the looming collapse of the climate and the natural world as we know it, my Heart wisdom tells me to follow in the footsteps of these ancient seers, to turn away from the deteriorating, deficient, rational modes of consciousness currently dominating our planet and open to another deeper, older and newer level of knowing. Here in the mystery of the unknown, the unpredictable, the imaginal, I find my way back to a light that can actually guide me through the turmoil as a new possibility for being human emerges from the chaos.

Moving aside the magic, the dreams, the beauty, I would like to share some of the decisions and practical steps that have helped me see "heaven's scatterings of stardust" in the world around me and actually access the spirit of the acupuncture points in the treatment room. Then I would like to offer some safe, practical ways you can integrate this kind of alchemical work into your current programs or practices.

Bringing Spirit into the Treatment Room

Presence

This work is an alchemical meditation that requires my time, commitment and ongoing participation. I generally am first aware of a palpable sense of spirit entering the room when I slow down, feel my feet on the ground, pause, breathe and do whatever I can to be present and sincerely interested.

Sight

The light of the spirit responds to my sight. If I can see and recognize the flickering of the *shen* as a patient talks to me about their issues, tells me their story or rests on my treatment table, then this ephemeral light becomes part of the encounter. In most cases, the patient too becomes aware of a warmth, an opening, a release, an insight, a shift as if a part of them has returned. This special kind of "sight" requires that I keep my eyes soft and receptive but that I don't go to "sleep" or zone out—even when it seems not much is happening. Carefully tracking a patient's facial expression, color, voice tone, light in the eyes, pulse, breath and posture helps me to track the comings and goings of the *shen*.

Care

My deep, ongoing devotion and care for the spirits is what encourages them to settle down into the body: the spark of *shen* to nest in the Heart; the mists of the *hun* to deliver their dreams to the Liver; the *yi* to hold steady and bring possibility into form; the buried radiance of the *po* to illuminate the deepest levels of somatic wisdom; the light seed of the *zhi* to take root in the Kidneys.

Investigation and Research

In addition to honing my skills as a magician and seer, my work with the spirits also requires rigorous investigation, research and reflection. Exploring the etymology of the acupuncture points has been a way for me to sit at the feet of the great ancient physicians who, with clear intentionality and care, gave each point its own key—its own name. The Chinese characters for me are like ancient alchemical vessels I can open linguistically, through enlivened sight, in order to access their wisdom. Reading myths, studying symbols and understanding the language of dreams has also supported me in this aspect of the work. Last but not least, for the past three decades, I have heeded the admonition of my earliest mentor, J. R. Worsley, who told his students to "make nature your first and most important teacher." Following in the footsteps of the ancient Taoist poets and alchemists, I spend many hours watching the Ways of the Water, the Wood, the Fire, the Earth and the Metal in the world around me.

Practice

All alchemy relies on ongoing, devoted practice and *nei dan* or inner work. Find an inner work practice that you enjoy and make it a part of your life. Any moving meditation practice like *qi gong*, yoga, standing meditation, 5Rhythms dance, Quoya[4] or Feldenkrais will help you to open your embodied sensory perception to the flowing of qi and the dance of the *shen*. Watch your dreams and pay attention to the images that come to you from the stars. Meditate outdoors in nature on a regular basis, honoring the turning seasons with conscious ritual. And always do your own psycho-spiritual healing work before you ask your patients to do theirs with you. Your inner work will lead to graceful, easeful outer changes in your practice.

Trust

Last but not least, trust what you see and what you know from your own body-felt sense. It has taken me over three decades of practice to be ready to write this book, to stand for the miraculous that is hidden in the folds of our everyday lives and the magic that impregnates the wand of my needle. If you stay with these steps and practices, you too will discover your own unique magic and alchemy and you too will become a poet of points.

Strategies for Integration

My suggestion is that you spend at least a year with this book. Work with the various sections during their related seasons. For each season, pick an archetype, a single point, flower essence and oil and work with it on yourself. From an alchemical perspective, we can only discover the truth through our own embodied experience, so get to know the tools through your own sensory experience before offering them to others.

You do not have to change your whole practice to bring the spirit of the points into the clinical encounter. A spirit point can be a way to open or close a piece of work. Or it can be used to "tattoo" an insight, a hard-earned behavior change, a new commitment or life transformation into the skin of the subtle body. In fact, as you become more comfortable with working with the spirit points, a single point may be all a person needs on a given day.

Ask permission of the patient as well as of the point. The first time you bring in the spirit level to a therapeutic encounter, let your patient know that you will be touching the qi in a different way—touching the finest, most ephemeral level of vibration. Explain why and how the work may be different. And when you approach the point, bring the same courtesy and care. Don't assume the point is ready for this level of penetration. Rather, bring your fingertip and present awareness to the point and wait for a moment to see if it welcomes your touch. A breath at that moment is like a prayer before the needle goes in in search of the light.

Create your own point palette. Use the writings and reflections in this book as a jumping-off point, not an endpoint! Then, each season, pick a single new point that you feel called to know deeply. Follow the rabbit hole down as deep as it will take you through etymology, poetry, research and exploration on your own body. This is how you gain true mastery and ownership of the spirit of the points.

Remember that each of us is a microcosm of a macrocosmic reality. Heaven and Earth are within me. Each time we reignite the light of the *shen* in a patient's body, we are helping in some small way to reignite the light of soul and spirit on our planet.

Above and beyond all, let your own spirits shine!

January 1, 2020, New Year's Day

Spirit Points by Season

Winter: Water Spirit Points

- Bladder 1 - Eyes Bright - *Jing Ming*
- Bladder 47 (or 52) - Ambition Room - *Zhi Shi*
- Bladder 58 - Fly and Scatter - *Fei Yang*
- Bladder 60 - Kunlun Mountain - *Kunlun*
- Bladder 67 - Extremity of Yin - *Zhi Yin*
- Kidney 1 - Bubbling Spring - *Yong Guan*
- Kidney 3 - Greater Mountain Stream - *Tai Xi*
- Kidney 7 - Returning Current - *Fu Liu*
- Kidney 16 - Vitals Transfer Point - *Huang Shu*
- Kidney 25 - Spirit Storehouse - *Shen Cang*

Spring: Wood Spirit Points

- Gall Bladder 13 - Root of the Spirit - *Ben Shen*
- Gall Bladder 16 - Window of the Eye - *Mu Chuang*
- Gall Bladder 24 - Sun and Moon - *Ri Yue*
- Gall Bladder 37 - Bright and Clear - *Guang Ming*
- Gall Bladder 41 - Foot Above Tears - *Zu Lin Qi*
- Liver 3 - Supreme Rushing - *Tai Chong*
- Liver 5 - Insect Ditch - *Li Gou*
- Liver 8 - Crooked Spring - *Qu Quan*

- Liver 13 - Chapter Gate - *Zhang Men*
- Liver 14 - Gate of Hope - *Qi Men*

Summer: Fire Spirit Points

- Heart 1 - Utmost Source - *Ji Quan*
- Heart 7 - Spirit Gate - *Shen Men*
- Heart 8 - Lesser Mansion - *Shao Fu*
- Small Intestine 7 - Upright Branch - *Zhi Zheng*
- Small Intestine 19 - Listening Palace - *Ting Gong*
- Pericardium 8 - Palace of Weariness - *Lao Gong*
- Pericardium 9 - Rushing into the Middle - *Zhong Chong*
- Triple Heater 5 - Outer Frontier Gate - *Wai Guan*
- Conception Vessel 15 - Dove Tail - *Jiu Wei*
- Bladder 38 (or 43) - Rich for the Vitals - *Gao Huang Shu*

Late Summer: Earth Spirit Points

- Stomach 8 - Head Tied - *Tou Wei*
- Stomach 12 - Broken Bowl - *Que Pen*
- Stomach 25 - Celestial Pivot - *Tian Shu*
- Stomach 40 - Abundant Splendor - *Feng Long*
- Stomach 44 - Inner Courtyard - *Nei Ting*
- Spleen 3 - Supreme White - *Tai Bai*
- Spleen 5 - Merchant Mound - *Shang Qiu*
- Spleen 8 - Earth Motivator - *Di Ji*
- Spleen 9 - Yin Mound Spring - *Yin Ling Quan*
- Spleen 21 - Great Enveloping - *Da Bao*

Autumn: Metal Spirit Points

- Lung 1 - Middle Palace - *Zhong Fu*

- Lung 2 - Cloud Gate - *Yun Men*

- Lung 3 - Palace of Heaven - *Tian Fu*

- Lung 8 - Meridian Gutter - *Jing Qu*

- Lung 9 - Supreme Abyss - *Tai Yuan*

- Lung 10 - Fish Region - *Yu Ji*

- Large Intestine 5 - Yang Stream - *Yang Xi*

- Large Intestine 6 - Veering Passage - *Pian Li*

- Large Intestine 11 - Pool at the Crook - *Qu Chi*

- Large Intestine 18 - Support and Rush Out - *Fu Tu*

- Large Intestine 20 - Welcome Fragrance - *Ying Xiang*

- Bladder 42 (or 37) - Door of the Corporeal Soul - *Po Hu*

Application of Spirit Point Tools

Needles

In spirit-level treatment, less is usually more. At this level, the needle is like a magic wand that is able to touch and affect the finest, most ephemeral aspect of the qi, an invisible yet still very real aspect of our being. It is important to remember that unnecessarily strong needle *de qi* on spirit points can actually scatter rather than settle the *shen* and can have a traumatizing effect on the subtle body. Experiment with using needles with a finer gauge and remove the needle once you perceive change in the patient's pulse, breath, complexion and attitude.

Moxa

Spirits love Fire! Moxa is a good consideration for spirit points except when a patient is already overheated. Direct rice grain moxa activates the spirit of the point and can function to settle as well as activate the *shen* depending on the needs of the patient. Indirect pole moxa is a good alternative if a gentler, more gradual warmth is preferred.

Flower Essences

Flower essences contain the vibrational or soul imprint of the plants they were created from but almost no material residue of the plant itself. They were first developed in Dr. Edward Bach, an English bacteriologist, pathologist and homeopath, in the 1930s. Dr. Bach originally developed a repertory of 38 remedies that addressed basic issues of the body, mind and spirit. Today there are hundreds of other essences that have been developed by practitioners around the world and we can create our own from the plants that grow in our own particular environment.

Flower essences can be viewed as the quintessential spirit-level remedy, as most are made from flower blossoms, the part of plants related most closely to the Fire Element and to the *shen* or spirit. Many essences are produced by shining sunlight through the plant material as it floats in a bowl of water and thus sequestering the plant-activated light in a material substance.

Flower essences are gentle yet powerful allies to patients at every stage of the healing process. They are safe for patients of any age and level of health or illness. They are non-toxic, have no side effects, are not habit forming and do not interfere with any other medications or treatments. There are many ways they can be used and only a few caveats that should be observed when considering them.

- Take care not to let the glass applicator touch skin—dip the applicator in alcohol to clean it if it touches the skin.

- If the patient is alcohol-sensitive, essence can be dropped in a bit of boiling water to evaporate the alcohol before taking it. There are also essences that are preserved in glycerin rather than alcohol. In addition, a company called Tree Frog Farm produces flower essences preserved in red shiso and organic vinegar.

- Negative treatment responses are rare. In general, when the remedy is "not right" for the patient, there is little or no response to the treatment. If there is no change after two weeks, a remedy should be discontinued and another one suggested.

- It is important to stay in communication with patients while they are using the flower essences, as the relationship between patient, practitioner and flower is an important part of the alchemy.

For the purpose of spirit-point treatment, I apply a few drops of the essence undiluted directly to the point. I use a Q-tip or cotton ball or, if possible, simply apply from the dropper. Once the essence is on the point, press lightly with a finger or cotton ball and hold it for a minute or two so that it can be absorbed into the meridian. Encourage the patient to rest quietly for a few minutes to allow the essence to begin its work.

In addition, flower essences can be diluted at 2–4 drops in 4–6 oz water—and applied with a cotton ball to an entire meridian. Apply the essence and allow the patient to rest for ten minutes. The essence and point will join vibrations and change will be initiated.

Flower essences can also be taken internally after the treatment to deepen and enhance the effects. This allows patients to continue the work in between sessions. The protocol is simple:

- Fill a 30 ml dropper bottle with spring water.

- Add 3–7 drops of chosen remedy and add 1 tablespoon of brandy to preserve it.

- Take under the tongue at least four times a day, with four drops each time.

- Take the flower essence daily for two to three weeks and then re-evaluate the situation. Depending on patient's response, make changes as necessary.

Recommended for further study: Bellows, W. and Craydon, D. (2005) *Floral Acupuncture: Applying the Flower Essences of Dr. Bach to Acupuncture Sites*. Berkeley/Toronto: The Crossing Press.

Essential Oils

Essential oils are another powerful tool to consider when working at the spirit level. If certain guidelines are followed, oils are a safe way to deepen and enhance the effects of a treatment.

Essential oils are more yin than flower essences. This means they are heavier, have more residue of the base material and are less volatile. While flower essences enter our being directly at the light or spirit level, essential oils vibrate at a lower frequency and tend to activate the mental/emotional or soul level of being.

Although essential oils, when correctly administered, are non-toxic, safe and have relatively few negative side effects, they must be used with great care. Improper use can result in dermatitis, nausea and allergic responses. These are powerful, fast-acting medicinals with strong personalities that call for respect and wisdom!

There are a few basic safety guidelines for using essential oils.

- Do not take essential oils internally.

- Except in specific, supervised situations, do not apply essential oils directly to skin.

- Always discuss the oil with patients the first time it is used. Ask about allergies or environmental sensitivities.

- Go slow and err on the side of caution. Use extra caution during pregnancy and postpartum when women are particularly sensitive to fragrance. Uterine stimulant oils such as angelica must be avoided during pregnancy.

For the purpose of spirit-level acupuncture treatment, a drop or two of undiluted oil is applied directly to the point with a Q-tip, cotton ball or fingertip. It is important to give the oil time to be absorbed through the skin and enter the meridian. One drop on a Q-tip can be applied before needling or held in place for a few minutes as an alternative to needling. Using the oil as an alternative to needles is useful for children or patients who are very sensitive to needling.

In addition to direct application, there are other ways that oils can be brought into the treatment process.

- Direct palm inhalation: A few drops of oil are sprinkled on the palms, which are rubbed together and offered for inhalation or used to massage the back of the neck and shoulders. This method is safe for oils that do not have a strong irritant effect.

- Massage and body oils: The best carriers are coconut, jojoba and sesame oil, although check that the patient is not sensitive to any of these. Use a 2–4% dilution or dilute until the correct level of fragrance is achieved.

- Bath: This is a wonderful way for patients to continue treatment at home, but it is important not to drop oil directly into the bath water, where it will collect in droplets and possibly irritate the skin. Essential oil can be emulsified with milk or honey or dispersed into salt. In this way, it will diffuse evenly into the bath water and be safe for the skin. The doses used for aromatic baths is very low, in the range of 5–10 drops depending on the oil.

- Aromatherapy: 5–10 drops of oil added to a half ounce of carrier oil can be given to patients to use at home. Application to specific points can be suggested or the oil can be inhaled as needed.

- Steam inhalation: 2–4 drops of oil in a basin of hot water. Form a tent with a towel over the head and inhale.

Recommended for further study: Mojay, G. (1997) *Aromatherapy: Healing the Spirit*. Rochester: Healing Arts Press.

Other Tools

Anything that stirs the qi can be used as a tool when touching the spirit level of a point. When used in conjunction with needle stimulation, or on their own, conscious inclusion of these tools in a clinical encounter can make the difference between a good session that helps a patient feel better physically and a session that touches the soul.

- Language, story, myth, metaphor and poetry.

- Visualization: Use the imagery of the point names to activate the imagination.

- Clear intention.

- Conscious touch: How you locate and touch the point matters to the spirit.

- Deep listening.

- Bringing the elements and the gifts of the seasons into the treatment room.

Understanding Chinese Characters

The Chinese language is not an alphabet language but rather a pictographic language made up of visual symbols called characters. The written characters traditionally had a spiritual significance for the ancient Chinese who believed that they had a Divine origin. In fact, one mythical explanation of the origins of the Chinese language is that the characters first came to the Yellow Emperor in the form of cloud scrolls from Heaven.

In order to grasp the spirit-level meaning of the point names, I find that it is important to meditate not only on their poetry but also on the wisdom contained in the graphic design and energetics of the original Chinese characters. You don't have to be a scholar or a sinologist to explore the characters that make up the point names, but there are a few things you do need to know about the Chinese language in order to begin your investigation.

The character is a graphic depiction of an energetic or a physical phenomenon. The graphic meaning of some characters is quite obvious. The character for tree 木 *mu* is quite clearly a picture of a tree with branches reaching outwards and roots sinking down into the ground. Mountain 山 *shan* is a clear, if somewhat abstracted, image of a mountain. In other cases, the graphic link is not so direct. For example, the word for acupuncture point 穴 *xue* takes more time to figure out, but if you stay with it, something emerges.

All Chinese characters are formed from seven simple strokes made up of dots and lines. The strokes come together to form the shape symbols that are the building blocks of the language. These basic building blocks are called radicals. A single word or character may be made up of anywhere between one and four radicals.

In general, one of the radicals that makes up a character gives us a clue to the meaning. This radical is called the semantic component. Another of the radicals, called the phonetic, gives us a clue to the verbal pronunciation of the word but may also, secondarily, add to our understanding of the word's deeper meaning.

Most point names are made up of two characters although there are a few that are made up of three. The names have multiple levels of meaning. The first level is often a reference to an aspect of the point's anatomical location. The second level may have to do with its physical effect. However, at the deepest level, the name gives us a clue to the hidden spirit: the point's capacity to touch the soul and move us on a path of transformation. At this deep level, the point name is a riddle waiting to be deciphered, a poem waiting to be heard, a message hidden in a bottle that has been waiting thousands of years for you to open it!

Resources for Further Learning

- Lindqvist, C. (Tate, J. trans.) (2008) *China: Empire of Living Symbols*. Reading: Addison-Wesley Publishing. (Original work published 1991.)

- Wenlin Institute. *Wenlin Software for Learning Chinese*, see: https://wenlin.com

Resources

Flower Essences

Flower Essence Services
P.O. Box 1769
Nevada City, CA 95959
800-548-0075
info@flowersociety.org
www.fesflowers.com

Healing Herbs Ltd.
Walterstone
Hereford HR2 0DX
United Kingdom
01873 890218
info@healingherbs.co.uk
www.healingherbs.co.uk

Oceans and Rivers (Essentials flower essence blends)
Sacred Studio
197 Clifton Place
Brooklyn, NY 11205
718-913-0037
lindsay@oceansandrivers.com
www.oceansandrivers.com

Nelson Bach USA, Ltd.
21 High Street, Suite 302
North Andover, MA 01845
800-319-9151
USACustomerService@nelsons.net
www.nelsons.net

Tree Frog Farm (offers essences with brandy base or non-alcoholic red shiso leaf base)
3679 Sunrise Road
Lummi Island, WA 98262
360-758-7260
info@treefrogfarm.com
www.treefrogfarm.com

Wonderworks
25 Baldwin Street
Toronto, ON M5T 1L1
Canada
416-323-3131
800-329-0757 (international)
www.gowonderworks.com

Essential Oils

Essential Therapeutics
39 Melverton Drive
Hallam, Victoria 3803
Australia
03 8795 7720
www.essentialtherapeutics.com.au

Floracopeia
13100 Grass Valley Avenue, Suite D
Grass Valley, CA 95945
866-417-1149
support@floracopeia.com
www.floracopeia.com

Original Swiss Aromatics
P.O. Box 6842
San Rafael, CA 94903
415-479-9120
www.originalswissaromatics.com

References

Balkin, J. (trans. and commentary) (2002) *The Laws of Change: I Ching and the Philosophy of Life*. Branford: Sybil Creek Press.

Barks, C. (trans. and commentary) (1997) *The Illuminated Rumi*. New York: Broadway Books.

Bellows, W. and Craydon, D. (2005) *Floral Acupuncture: Applying the Flower Essences of Dr. Bach to Acupuncture Sites*. Berkeley/Toronto: The Crossing Press.

Cahill, S. (1993) *Transcendence and Divine Passion: The Queen Mother of the West in Medieval China*. Stanford: Stanford University Press.

Deadman, P. and Al-Khafaji, M. with Baker, K. (1998) *A Manual of Acupuncture*. Hove: Journal of Chinese Medicine Publications.

Dechar, L. E. (2006) *Five Spirits: Alchemical Acupuncture for Psychological and Spiritual Healing*. New York: Chiron Publications/Lantern Books.

Dechar, L. E. with Fox, B. (2019) *The Alchemy of Inner Work*. Newburyport: Red Wheel Weiser Conari Publishers.

Dharmananda, S. (2004) *Ma Danyang's Twelve Acupoints: Valuable Points for Acupuncturists to Know and Use*. Portland: Institute for Traditional Medicine. Accessed on 9/15/19 at www.itmonline.org/arts/madanyang.htm.

Hertzer, D. (2009) 'Talk on the *Xiuzhen Tu*.' Second Annual TCM Kongress in Denmark, September 2009. (Personal transcription.)

Hinton, D. (2016) *Existence: A Story*. Boulder: Shambhala Publications.

Jung, C. (1990) *The Archetypes of the Collective Unconscious*. Princeton: Bollingen Press. (Original work published 1959.)

Kaatz, D. (2005) *Characters of Wisdom: Taoist Tales of the Acupuncture Points*. Soudorgues: Petite Bergerie Press.

Larre, C. and Rochat de la Vallée, E. (1998) *Heart Master Triple Heater.* Cambridge: Monkey Press.

Larre, C. and Rochat de la Vallée, E. (2001) *The Lung.* Cambridge: Monkey Press.

Larre, C. and Rochat de la Vallée, E. (2003) *The Secret Treatise of the Spiritual Orchid: Nei Jing Su Wen Chapter 8.* Cambridge: Monkey Press.

Larre, C., Schatz, J. and Rochat de la Vallée, E. (trans. and commentary) (Stang, S. trans.) (1986) *Survey of Traditional Chinese Medicine.* Paris: Institut Ricci.

Kaminski, P. and Katz, R. (1994) *Flower Essence Repertory: A Comprehensive Guide to North American and English Flower Essences for Emotional and Spiritual Well-Being.* Nevada City: The Flower Essence Society.

Kohn, L. (ed.) (1996) *The Taoist Experience.* Albany: State University of New York.

Lindqvist, C. (Tate, J. trans.) (2008) *China: Empire of Living Symbols.* Reading: Addison-Wesley Publishing. (Original work published 1991.)

Mojay, G. (1997) *Aromatherapy: Healing the Spirit.* Rochester: Healing Arts Press.

Nugent-Head, A. (2012) 'The Heavenly Star Points of Ma Danyang.' *Journal of Chinese Medicine 98,* 5–12.

Plaingam, W., Sangsuthum, S., Angkhasirisap, W. and Tencomnao, T. (2017) '*Kaempferia parviflora* rhizome extract and *Myristica fragrans* volatile oil increase the levels of monoamine neurotransmitters and impact the proteomic profiles in the rat hippocampus: Mechanistic insights into their neuroprotective effects.' *Journal of Traditional and Complementary Medicine 7,* 4 538–552.

Pound, E. (1971) *Selected Poems.* London: Faber and Faber. (Original work published 1928.)

Preston, R. (2008) *The Wild Trees: A Story of Passion and Daring.* New York: Random House.

Rochat de la Vallée, E. (2009) *Wu Xing: The Five Elements in Chinese Classical Texts.* London: Monkey Press.

Ronnberg, A. (ed.) (2010) *The Book of Symbols: Reflections on Archetypal Images.* Cologne: Taschen Press.

Star, J. (trans.) (2001) *Tao Te Ching: The Definitive Edition.* New York: Tarcher.

Tokutomi, K. (1993) *Kigo and Form: The World of Kigo.* San Jose: Yuki Tekei Haiku Society. Accessed on 9/22/19 at https://youngleaves. org/?page_id=105.

Tolkien, J. R. R. (2012) *The Fellowship of the Ring.* New York: Houghton Mifflin Harcourt. (Original work published 1937.)

Twicken, D. (2013) *Eight Extraordinary Channels: Qi Jong Ba Mai.* London: Singing Dragon.

Veith, I. (trans.) (2015) *The Yellow Emperor's Class of Internal Medicine.* Berkeley: University of California Press. (Original work published 1972.)

Warwick, T. (ed.) (2015) *The Rosary of the Philosophers.* Middletown: Tari Warwick. (Original work published 1550.)

Watson, B. (trans.) (1977) *Ryokan: Zen Monk-Poet of Japan.* New York: Columbia University Press.

Watts, A. (1975) *Tao: The Watercourse Way.* New York: Pantheon Books.

Wenlin Institute (2007) *Wenlin Software for Learning Chinese.* Version 3.4.1.

Wilhelm, R. (trans.) (1942) *The Secret of the Golden Flower: A Chinese Book of Life.* London: Kegan Paul, Trench, Trubner & Co.

Wilhelm, R. (trans.) (1983) *The I Ching or Book of Changes.* Princeton: Princeton University Press. (Original work published 1950.)

Willmont, D. (2004) *The Twelve Spirit Points of Acupuncture.* Marshfield: Willmountain Press. (Original work published 1999.)

Worsley, J.R. (1998) *The Five Elements and the Officials.* Leamington Spa: College of Traditional Acupuncture.

Wu, J. (trans.) (1961) *Lao Tzu: Tao Teh Ching.* New York: St. John's University Press.

Yuasa, N. (trans.) (1967) *Basho: The Narrow Road to the Deep North.* New York: Penguin Books.

Bibliography

Aria, B. with Eng Gon, R. (1992) *The Spirit of the Chinese Character: Gifts from the Heart.* San Francisco: Chronicle Books.

Blome, G., M.D. (1999) *Advanced Bach Flower Therapy: A Scientific Approach to Diagnosis and Treatment.* Rochester: Healing Arts Press.

Ellis, A., Wiseman, N. and Boss, K. (1991) *Fundamentals of Chinese Acupuncture.* Brookline: Paradigm Publishers.

Foster, N. and Shoemaker, J. (eds) (1996) *The Roaring Stream: A New Zen Reader.* Hopewell: Ecco Press.

Gilbert, R. (2005) *Kigo Versus Seasonal Reference in Haiku: Observations, Anecdotes and a Translation.* Simply Haiku, Autumn 3.3. Accessed on 9/15/19 at www.gendaihaiku.com/research/kigo/07-sh-kigo-and-seasonal-reference-2005.pdf.

Johnson, J. A. (2006) *Chinese Medical Qigong Therapy: A Comprehensive Clinical Text.* Pacific Grove: International Institute of Medical Qigong.

Kirkwood, J. (2016) *The Way of the Five Elements: 52 Weeks of Powerful Acupoints for Physical, Emotional, and Spiritual Health.* London: Singing Dragon.

Larre, C. and Rochat de la Vallée, E. (1995) *Rooted in Spirit: The Heart of Chinese Medicine.* Barrytown: Station Hill Press.

Larre, C. and Rochat de la Vallée, E. (1991) *The Heart in Lingshu Chapter 8.* Cambridge: Monkey Press.

Morgan, H. (1942) *Chinese Symbols and Superstitions.* South Pasadena: P. D. and Ione Perkins.

Pelikan, W. (Lebensart, C. trans.) (1973) *The Secret Life of Metals.* Great Barrington: Lindisfarne Books.

Powell, J. (1882) *The Tao of Symbols: How to Transcend the Limits of our Symbolism*. New York: William Morrow and Company.

Pregadio, F. (2019) *Xiuzhen Tu (Chart for the Cultivation of Reality)*. The Golden Elixir, Mountain View: Golden Elixir Press. Accessed on 9/15/10 at https://goldenelixir.com/jindan/xiuzhen_tu.html.

Schnaubelt, K. (2011) *The Healing Intelligence of Essential Oils*. Rochester: Healing Arts Press.

Stewart, H. (ed. and trans.) (1960) *A Net of Fireflies: Japanese Haiku and Haiku Paintings*. Rutland: Charles E. Tuttle Company.

Endnotes

Foreword

1. Dechar 2006

Introduction

2. Tokutomi 1993, p.1
3. Veith (trans.) 2015, first published 1972, p.149

Water: Winter Season

1. Wu (trans.) 1961, p.11
2. Veith (trans.) 2015, first published 1972, p.113
3. *Ibid.*, p.141
4. Worsley 1998, p.167
5. Veith (trans.) 2015, first published 1972, p.113
6. Neuroscientist Paul D. MacLean coined the term "reptilian brain" to refer to the basal ganglia structures, the most primal part of what he viewed as the triune or three-part human brain. He referred to this most ancient, earliest, evolving part of the nervous system as the "reptilian complex," as it is responsible for instinctual behaviors including aggression, dominance, territoriality and ritual displays that are common to all modern vertebrates.
7. Kohn 1996, p.56
8. *Ibid.*
9. Cahill 1993, p.48
10. Kohn 1996, p.59
11. Deadman, Al-Khafaji and Baker 1998, p.257

12. Kaatz 2005, p.446

13. *Ibid.*, p.446

14. Dechar and Fox 2019, p.176

15. Lindqvist 2008, first published 1991, p.78

16. Kaatz 2005, p.512

17. Mojay 1997, p.59

18. Dechar 2006, p.152

19. Balkin 2002, p.511

20. Ma Yu, who later took the name Ma Danyang (Yang Cinnabar or Yang Alchemy), was born to a wealthy family in Shandong Province and showed early talents as both an acupuncturist and a poet. He married one of most revered of the ancient women Taoist sages, Sun Bu'er, and together they left to become monks and live in retreat with Wang Chongyang, one of the leading Taoist teachers in China. The ode that is attributed to him may also have been written in part or dictated to him by his teacher, Wang.

21. Dharmananda 2004

22. *Ibid.*

23. *Ibid.*

24. Plaingam *et al.* 2017

25. Deadman, Al-Khafaji and Baker 1998, p.318

26. Lindqvist 2008, first published 1991, p.78

27. Kaatz 2005, p.512

28. Deadman, Al-Khafaji and Baker 1998, p.336

29. Wilhelm (trans.) 1983, first published 1950, p.97

30. *Ibid.*, p.97

31. *Ibid.*, p.139

32. *Ibid.*, p.140

Wood: Spring Season

1. Pound 1971, first published 1928, p.95

2. Rochat de la Vallée 2009, p.70

3. Veith (trans.) 2015, first published 1972, p.112

4. *Ibid.*, p.141

5. *Ibid.*, p.118

6. Ronnberg (ed.) 2010, p.10

7. Wilhelm (trans.) 1983, first published 1950, p.3

8. *Ibid.*, pp.7–10

9. *Ibid.*, p.9

10. *Ibid.*

11. *Ibid.*, p.10

12. Preston 2008, p.277

13. Tolkien 2012, first published 1937, p.147

14. *Ibid.*

15. Twicken 2013, p.103

16. Deadman, Al-Khafaji and Baker 1998, p.434

17. Kaatz 2005, p.187

18. Mojay 1997, p.62

19. Deadman, Al-Khafaji and Baker 1998, p.442

20. *Ibid.*, p.434

21. *Ibid.*, p.454

22. Wilhelm 1983, first published 1950, p.79

23. *Ibid.*

24. *Ibid.*

25. Twicken 2013, p.138

26. See entry and notes for Bladder 60 - Kunlun Mountain - *Kunlun* for more information on Ma Danyang and the Twelve Heavenly Star Points.

27. Dharmananda 2004

28. *Ibid.*

29. Deadman, Al-Khafaji and Baker 1998, p.478

30. Star (trans.) 2001, p.21

31. *Ibid.*, p.65

Fire: Summer Season

1. Star (trans.) 2001, p.119

2. The close correlation between the sound of the Chinese character for *huo* 火 Fire and *hua* 花 flower and the fact that both characters are associated with the idea of transformation confirms their linguistic and symbolic connection.

3. Veith (trans.) 2015, first published 1972, p.112

4. *Ibid.*, p.141

5. *Ibid.*, p.134

6. Worsley 1998, p.137

7. Wu 1961, p.23

8. Larre and Rochat de la Vallée 1998, p.2

9. Veith (trans.) 2015, first published 1972, p.133

10. Larre and Rochat de la Vallée 1998, p.51

11. Worsley 1998, p.123

12. Larre and Rochat de la Vallée 1998, pp.8–12

13. Larre and Rochat de la Vallée 2003, p.119

14. Veith (trans) 2015, first published 1972, p.133

15. *Ibid.*, p.222

16. For more on the alchemical nature of cinnabar, see Dechar 2006, pp.100–102

17. Warwick (ed.) 2015, first published 1550, p.157–158

18. Jung 1990, first published 1959, p.164

19. From a personal transcription of a talk on the *Xiuzhen Tu* by Dominique Hertzer at the Second Annual TCM Kongress in Denmark, September 2009.

20. *Ibid.*

21. Barks (trans.) 1997, p.68

22. *Ibid.*

23. Ronnberg (ed), 2010, p.394

24. Dechar 2006, p.175

25. The word "appropriate" is used here in the Taoist sense to refer to actions and timing that are in alignment with Tao as opposed to the Western use of the word to indicate collective expectations and social norms.

26. Ronnberg (ed.) 2010, p.162

27. Deadman, Al-Khafaji and Baker 1998, p.221

28. Mojay 1997, p.117

29. Deadman, Al-Khafaji and Baker 1998, p.238

30. Kaminski and Katz 1994, p.399

31. This variant on the meaning of the word *gong* as womb or uterus circles back to the Chinese word for Pericardium *xin bao* 心包, literally translated as heart wrapper, and affirms our understanding of the Pericardium's function as semi-permeable membrane and Heart Protector. The radical *bao* 勹 is a picture of a wrapping that surrounds a *si* 巳 fetus so the Pericardium can be understood as a kind of womb that encloses and protects the Heart.

32. Sun Simiao recognized that these 13 points had powerful effects on the psycho-emotional states of his patients. In particular, he noted their capacity to clear phlegm that was misting the heart, impeding a person's clear thought and blocking their ability to know and live from their own true nature.

33. Deadman, Al-Khafaji and Baker 1998, p.50

34. Larre and Rochat de la Vallée 1998, p.3

35. *Ibid.*, p.51

36. Deadman, Al-Khafaji and Baker 1998, p.396

37. *Ibid.*, p.516

38. Willmont 2004, p.41

39. Deadman, Al-Khafaji and Baker 1998, p.516

40. This viscous, sticky accumulated substance could be considered to be an aspect of what is now diagnosed as atherosclerotic disease.

41. Deadman, Al-Khafaji and Baker 1998, p.303

42. See Deadman, Al-Khafaji and Baker 1998, p.303, quoting classic texts on the significance of the *gau huang* and the inestimable value of this point from Zuo-jiu 501 BCE through Sun Simiao in 1360 AD.

43. Deadman, Al-Khafaji and Baker 1998, p.304

44. *Ibid.*

Earth: Late Summer Season

1. Veith (trans.) 2015, first published 1972, p.112

2. *Ibid.*, p.141

3. *Ibid.*, p.109

4. Worsley 1998, p.143

5. The *dan tian* refers to the lower abdomen where the organs of digestion, excretion and reproduction are located. In inner alchemy, these organs are considered vessels of transformation. This is the area focused on in many *qi gong* and meditation practices as it is the place where vital life energies can be cultivated.

6. Watts 1975, p.107

7. Watson (trans.) 1977, p.29

8. *Ibid.*, p.30

9. *Ibid.*, p.27

10. The ancient Chinese myth of creation describes the original universe as a swirling chaos. This primordial chaotic state eventually coalesced into an enormous egg. Within the egg, the opposed principles of yin and yang became balanced, and the giant, Pan Gu, the creator of the manifest universe, was conceived. Over the course of 18,000 years, Pan Gu grew too large for the egg. At that point, he smashed the shell, emerged from the egg and began creating the world.

11. Wilhelm (trans.) 1983, first published 1950, p.214

12. Dharmananda 2004, p.1

13. Nugent-Head 2012, p.9

14. Dharmananda 2004, p.2

15. Nugent-Head 2012, p.7

16. Deadman, Al-Khafaji and Baker 1998, p.188

17. Kaatz 2005, p.377

18. Worsley 1998, p.38

19. *Ibid.*

20. Deadman, Al-Khafaji and Baker 1998, p.204

Metal: Autumn Season

1. Rochat de la Vallée 2009, p.71

2. Veith (trans.) 2015, first published 1972, p.112

3. *Ibid.*, p.141

4. *Neijing Suwen*, translated and quoted in Larre and Rochat de la Vallée 2001, p.96

5. *Ibid.*, p.206

6. Worsley 1998, p.153

7. Larre and Rochat de la Vallée 2001, p.17

8. Jung 1990, first published 1959, p. 29

9. This can also be translated as "Po Door."

10. Deadman, Al-Khafaji and Baker 1998, p.48

Conclusion: Scattering Stardust

1. Barks (trans) 1997, p.99

2. Hinton 2016, p.6

3. *Ibid.*, p.7

4. Quoya is a movement system based on the idea that through movement, we remember and can learn to trust the physical sensation of truth in our bodies.

Index

Note: Illustrations are indicated by page numbers given in *italics*